Managing
Type 2 Diabetes

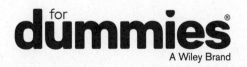

A Wiley Brand

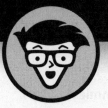

Managing Type 2 Diabetes

by American Diabetes Association®

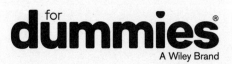

A Wiley Brand

Managing Type 2 Diabetes For Dummies®

Published by: **John Wiley & Sons, Inc.,** 111 River Street, Hoboken, NJ 07030-5774, www.wiley.com

Copyright © 2018 by John Wiley & Sons, Inc., Hoboken, New Jersey

Published simultaneously in Canada

For general information on our other products and services, please contact our Customer Care Department within the U.S. at 877-762-2974, outside the U.S. at 317-572-3993, or fax 317-572-4002. For technical support, please visit https://hub.wiley.com/community/support/dummies.

Wiley publishes in a variety of print and electronic formats and by print-on-demand. Some material included with standard print versions of this book may not be included in e-books or in print-on-demand. If this book refers to media such as a CD or DVD that is not included in the version you purchased, you may download this material at http://booksupport.wiley.com. For more information about Wiley products, visit www.wiley.com.

Library of Congress Control Number: 2017961517

ISBN 978-1-119-36329-3 (pbk); ISBN 978-1-119-36330-9 (ebk); ISBN 978-1-119-36331-6 (ebk)

Manufactured in the United States of America

10 9 8 7 6 5 4 3 2 1

Contents at a Glance

Table of Contents

Introduction

Diabetes touches everyone. You may have diabetes, or you may take care of a loved one like a parent, spouse, or teen with this chronic condition. It's incredibly personal, and yet it's global. According to the World Health Organization, 422 million people around the world had diabetes in 2014. That's a whopping 8.5 percent of the earth's population.

Largely, diabetes is a condition that you manage on your own. In other words, you're the top dog. You're the person in charge of your care. There's even a name for it: self-care. You're responsible for learning about diabetes, assembling a healthcare team, taking steps to exercise and eat healthy, and discovering how to manage and treat your blood glucose. Yet, you may have been diagnosed with diabetes for reasons out of your control, such as a family history or because your race and ethnicity put you at higher risk for type 2 diabetes. The factors that contribute to each person's diagnosis of diabetes aren't always obvious.

Put in this context, diabetes is quite a journey for most of us. And it's almost always an opportunity to take better care of yourself because you're at the center of your healthcare. It can be empowering to realize that you're responsible for making choices that will impact your health today and for decades in the future.

About This Book

You're about to find out a lot about diabetes — at least enough to get started on this journey. You'll discover how to become a better healthcare consumer and take actionable steps to manage your diabetes and prevent complications. Of course, there are many books out there dedicated to diabetes, and we're thankful for all of them.

This book is focused solely on type 2 diabetes. We hope opening this book is like turning to a trusted friend or your favorite nurse to get answers to questions that you never had the time (or opportunity) to ask. There are no dumb questions in a *For Dummies* book.

This book was written by the American Diabetes Association, an organization dedicated to fighting diabetes and its deadly consequences through cutting-edge medical research, public health information, advocacy for people's rights with diabetes in the workplace and school, and more. This is a group of volunteers, members, healthcare professionals, and staff with the sole motivation to prevent and cure diabetes. We're on the front lines, right there with you.

This book is organized in easy-to-read parts that focus on specific topics such as how to get started, eating healthy, and staying active. Unlike the last novel you read, don't expect to read this book from front to back. Instead, think of this book as a reference. You can dip in and out of topics as they relate to your diagnosis, care, and questions or concerns. You won't find a pop quiz at the end, and frankly, remembering every detail isn't the point. Use this book as reference when taking care of your type 2 diabetes or someone you love with diabetes.

You can skip the Technical Stuff icons and sidebars if you don't need the nitty-gritty details on a particular topic. You're going to see reasonable recommendations that the American Diabetes Association makes for most people with diabetes. These are just guidelines. It's up to you and your healthcare provider to set your own goals for managing diabetes and preventing complications. Your goals should be based on your individual needs.

Within this book, you may note that some web addresses break across two lines of text. If you're reading this book in print and want to visit one of these web pages, simply key in the web address exactly as it's noted in the text, pretending as though the line break doesn't exist. If you're reading this as an e-book, you've got it easy — just click the web address to be taken directly to the web page.

Foolish Assumptions

If you're reading this book, you probably have diabetes or someone very close to you has diabetes. However, you may know almost nothing about diabetes because you've never had to deal with it before. Don't worry — this book is for you.

You may not have ever set eyes on a blood glucose meter or pricked your skin for a blood sample. Or perhaps you have a family of people who have type 2 diabetes — and now you find yourself with the same diagnosis. You may have thought that you knew certain things about diabetes, but now wonder if those assumptions are really true. It's time to find out.

Whatever your background, you'll discover the basics of diabetes and its impact on your body in this book. You don't even have to remember anything from your high school biology class to get started. You can use this information to understand why it's important to take care of your diabetes so you can feel good each day and live a long and healthy life free of complications. You'll find out how to build a healthcare team and ask the right questions during checkups. You'll discover the latest medications and technology for taking care of your type 2 diabetes. You'll learn the basic steps to take toward eating wholesome, nutritious foods and exercising more regularly. You may use this knowledge for yourself or use it to take care of someone you care about deeply.

Icons Used in This Book

Icons throughout the book alert you to helpful information, facts to remember, and technical information that may help if you're looking for a more advanced understanding of the topic.

TIP

This icon marks important information that can save you time or make your life easier.

REMEMBER

This icon flags important information. Commit it to your memory or mark it so you find it again for easy reference.

WARNING

This icon warns about potential problems — health related and other.

TECHNICAL STUFF

This icon gives you information that may be helpful, but it's not necessary to your understanding of the topic at hand.

Beyond the Book

In addition to the book you're reading right now, be sure to check out the free online Cheat Sheet for details on diabetes checkups, checking your blood glucose, treating low blood glucose, and reading food labels for carbohydrate. To get this Cheat Sheet, simply go to www.dummies.com and type **Type 2 Diabetes For Dummies** in the Search box.

Where to Go from Here

Turning this page to get started is a great next step in discovering what you need to know about diabetes. You're about to uncover the basics of type 2 diabetes, including the role of the pancreas, insulin, and blood glucose. *Remember:* This is the part where you *don't* need to remember anything about high school biology to jump right in. Perhaps more important, in Chapter 2 you find out why it's critical to take care of your diabetes. That knowledge and confidence can give you a foundation for taking many of the action steps described in the rest of the book.

What if you already know a lot about type 2 diabetes? What if you're already inspired to take charge of your health? Then feel free to skip to the chapter that most intrigues you. Perhaps it's a chapter on women's health or taking care of your mental health. Maybe you're eager to get more information about checking blood glucose or bariatric surgery. Take a look at the topic of each chapter and start with the one that's most important to your diabetes care.

Remember: Diabetes is a journey. You'll learn to live with it every day, and some days will be better than others. This book can help you on those days when you need a reference to troubleshoot a problem or make meaningful changes to your health.

1
Getting Started with Diabetes

IN THIS PART . . .

Find out the basics of diabetes, including how it affects your entire body, understand how diabetes is diagnosed, and discover the risk factors.

Uncover why it's important to take care of yourself — today and for the future — and take the first steps toward managing your diabetes by making healthy choices in your everyday life.

Chapter **1**

Type 2 Diabetes: The Basics

Taking care of your diabetes means taking care of your whole body: from positive thinking in your brain to checking the bottoms of your feet for scrapes and cuts. It's a whole-body endeavor, and we're here to take you on that journey as you discover what diabetes is, how to manage and treat it, and how to prevent complications down the road.

This chapter starts off with the basics of diabetes: what it is and how it affects your body. These are the Biology 101 facts that you can reference down the line. It's fascinating stuff (and you don't need a medical degree to understand it). Then we tell you who else has diabetes and what the contributing risk factors are. After all, you're not the only one with diabetes. As of 2015, more than 30 million people in the United States had it, too.

What Exactly Is Diabetes?

You have diabetes, or perhaps someone you love has diabetes. That's not an easy diagnosis to hear. But it doesn't have to be a scary unknown either. In fact, scientists know more about diabetes and have more tools at their disposal than ever before.

The following sections explain how diabetes affects your body. It's good to know what's happening before you dive into how to manage and treat diabetes.

Getting the lowdown on blood glucose

Diabetes is a disorder in which the amount of glucose, also called sugar, is too high in the blood. When you were diagnosed with type 2 diabetes, you were probably told that your blood glucose was sky high. But why would your blood glucose be high?

It all comes down to eating — that amazing topic that everyone likes to obsess about. When you eat food, your body breaks that food down into glucose, and then the glucose travels in your bloodstream to waiting cells. That glucose really wants to get out of your blood and into your cells because that's how you get energy. That's the goal!

Insulin is a hormone that helps move glucose from your blood to inside your cells. However, people with type 2 diabetes don't make enough insulin or aren't as sensitive to that hormone. Therefore, the glucose gets trapped in the blood and can't get inside your cells. Then high blood glucose — diabetes — happens.

TECHNICAL STUFF

Glucose is just a simple form of carbohydrate. The simplest carbohydrates are sugars, and the simplest sugar is glucose. It's your body's main source of energy, used to power everything from getting up in the morning to taking your dog for a walk. Is it blood glucose or blood sugar? Actually they're the same thing. Blood glucose is simple sugar. So, you may hear people say their "sugars" are too high or their blood glucose is too high. Blood glucose is the more technical term; sugar is the more colloquial term. We use *blood glucose*, or simply *glucose*, in this book.

The mighty hormone insulin

You've probably heard of insulin, and you may associate it with injections or an insulin pump. We usually think of that as the synthetic or man-made medication. But the hormone in your body is also insulin. And it's one of the most important hormones for helping you metabolize your food and get energy.

Specialized beta cells in the pancreas make insulin. The pancreas, which is totally essential and underappreciated (until it stops working), is little, about 6 inches long, and sits right behind your stomach (see Figure 1-1).

The pancreas has islet cells that include both beta cells, which make insulin, and alpha cells, which make another hormone called glucagon. Both insulin and glucagon are important for metabolizing food.

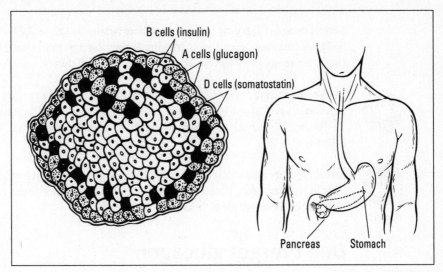

Illustration by Kathryn Born, MA

FIGURE 1-1:
The pancreas
and its
specialized cells.

Beta cells are the only cells that make insulin. In type 2 diabetes, several things are happening with those beta cells:

» **The beta cells don't work well.** They don't make as much insulin as they're supposed to.

» **There may be fewer beta cells than usual.**

» **The beta cells that are making all the insulin get burned out (super tired) and eventually make less insulin.** It's a cycle in which insulin production can get worse over time.

At the same time that beta cells are struggling in the pancreas, another crazy thing happens: Cells in your body become less sensitive to insulin. So, even though the insulin may be sitting right next to the glucose by a cell, saying, "Hey, let us in!" your cell doesn't let them in. Instead, your cells need more insulin than ever before to let those glucose molecules inside. This is called *insulin resistance* or *decreased insulin sensitivity.*

It's a double whammy: Your pancreas makes less insulin, and yet you need more insulin than ever before. It's not a good combination.

If your body doesn't make enough insulin or if you have insulin resistance, your glucose can't get inside your cells and builds up in your blood. This is called *high blood glucose.* It's the key factor that defines diabetes.

Scientists are still trying to figure out why beta cells fail or die — and also why the body becomes less sensitive to insulin. If they can get to the bottom of those questions, we're on our way toward a cure for type 2 diabetes.

TIP

In the meantime, scientists know that insulin sensitivity can be improved by exercise. Just a short bout of exercise can improve insulin sensitivity for up to 24 hours. It's another amazing effect of breaking a sweat besides burning calories.

REMEMBER

Insulin is a hormone that helps your cells use glucose for energy. It's made by beta cells in the pancreas. People with type 2 diabetes may not make enough insulin or may not be as sensitive to insulin — or both.

Don't forget glucagon

Your pancreas makes another hormone, glucagon, which works together with insulin to turn food into energy (refer to Figure 1-1). Glucagon works very closely with the liver by stimulating glucose stored inside it. This is an essential step when you need extra energy and you're not eating. For example, you might release glucagon when you exercise or if you need energy between meals. As you can see, it's a delicate balance to get energy from the foods you eat, but also have access to energy whenever you need it.

High blood glucose is not good

The bottom line is that people with type 2 diabetes have too much glucose in their blood.

High blood glucose can create problems in the short term and long term. It's so important because it can make you feel crummy from time to time, but it can also cause dangerous complications down the road.

As blood glucose levels rise, your body tries to flush out extra glucose in your blood by filtering it through your kidneys and out through your urine. That's why people with undiagnosed or out-of-control diabetes pee a lot. So much peeing causes people to feel thirsty, dehydrated, and tired. Dehydration can also blur vision.

However, high blood glucose may not cause these symptoms in everyone. Or sometimes the symptoms just aren't that noticeable. People can walk around for years without any symptoms or knowledge that they have high blood glucose and diabetes.

In the long term, high blood glucose damages blood vessels and nerves. The damage can lessen blood flow throughout your body, from your heart to your head to your feet. This, in turn, can lead to complications like eye disease, heart disease, stroke, and kidney failure. You find out more about complications in Chapter 8.

The great news is that you can take active steps to lower your blood glucose by eating wholesome foods, exercising, losing weight, and taking prescribed medications. You don't have to experience problems in the short or long term. The most important thing to remember is that you can take control of your blood glucose and diabetes.

Paying attention to blood pressure

Two out of every three people with diabetes have high blood pressure or take medications to lower it. That's a big number. Blood glucose and blood pressure go hand in hand. Why? Because they're both related to your blood vessels.

High blood glucose can damage blood vessels, causing them to narrow and inhibit the flow of blood. This in turn can cause high blood pressure, which can lead to further damage such as a heart attack, stroke, or kidney failure.

Also, diabetes and high blood pressure share similar risk factors, including smoking, obesity, and eating foods high in saturated fats. For example, if you're overweight and smoke cigarettes, it's a double whammy on your body.

WARNING

High blood pressure doesn't have any symptoms. You won't know you have high blood pressure until you have your blood pressure checked by your healthcare provider. Make sure you have it tested every time you visit your doctor or nurse.

Most people with diabetes will have a goal of less than 140 mmHg for systolic blood pressure (the top number) and less than 90 mmHg for diastolic blood pressure (the bottom number) to reduce the risk of cardiovascular disease and other complications.

Different Types of Diabetes

So far, you've heard all about type 2 diabetes, but there are actually many different types of diabetes. The most common type by far is type 2 diabetes. It accounts for 90–95 percent of all people with diabetes.

Type 1 diabetes

Type 1 diabetes is another common type of diabetes. It usually comes on much more severely than type 2 diabetes. In general, people with type 1 diabetes have to take insulin right away to survive because their bodies don't make any insulin. They have to take insulin for the rest of their lives. This is unlike type 2 diabetes, which has a more gradual progression.

Type 1 diabetes used to be called juvenile diabetes because it typically occurs in children. However, adults can also develop type 1 diabetes. Type 1 diabetes is an autoimmune disease in which the body destroys its own beta cells and, therefore, can no longer produce insulin. Of all the people with diabetes, about 5 percent have type 1 diabetes. (The "Type 1 or type 2?" sidebar explains how doctors determine whether you have type 1 or type 2 diabetes.)

Gestational diabetes

Gestational diabetes is a type of diabetes that occurs during pregnancy. It usually goes away after giving birth but gives moms and their babies a lifetime risk of developing type 2 diabetes. Women with gestational diabetes are more likely to someday have type 2 diabetes. Their children are also more likely to develop type 2 diabetes and be obese.

Women with gestational diabetes can take medications, eat healthy foods, and exercise to manage their blood glucose during pregnancy. Uncontrolled blood glucose during pregnancy can increase the risk of preeclampsia and injury during birth because babies are large. When you've had gestational diabetes, you have a two in three risk for it in subsequent pregnancies.

TYPE 1 OR TYPE 2?

Sometimes it's not obvious at first whether someone has type 1 or type 2 diabetes. A blood glucose test only tells you that you have diabetes, not whether it's type 1 or type 2 or some other form. For example, some adults may have type 1 diabetes, but still have some insulin production. This makes it appear more like type 2 diabetes at first. This is sometimes called *latent autoimmune diabetes* (LADA).

Your doctor can give you a separate test to help determine whether you have type 1 diabetes. People with type 1 diabetes have antibodies in their blood that signal an autoimmune disease. So, a physician can give you a blood test to detect autoantibodies and diagnose type 1 diabetes.

Gestational diabetes is different from already having type 2 diabetes and becoming pregnant. Women with preexisting type 2 diabetes should try to have their blood glucose on target before they become pregnant. They also need to exercise, eat healthy foods, and often take medications to manage their blood glucose during pregnancy.

TIP

All pregnant women should be tested for gestational diabetes during the 24th to 28th week using the oral glucose tolerance test (see Chapter 9 for more details on tests to diagnose gestational diabetes). Then women with gestational diabetes should get a test for type 2 diabetes 4–12 weeks after giving birth and every 3 years thereafter.

Other types of diabetes

Type 1, type 2, and gestational diabetes are the main types of diabetes. However, they're not the only ones. Other forms of diabetes occur because of mutations in single genes. You can inherit these gene mutations, or they can occur out of the blue. Maturity-onset diabetes of the young (MODY) and neonatal diabetes mellitus are two of the most common forms.

Cystic fibrosis–related diabetes is another type of diabetes common in people with cystic fibrosis, which occurs because of scarring of the pancreas. This also destroys beta cells and stops insulin production.

Prediabetes

Prediabetes is another term you've probably heard alongside type 2 diabetes. And it's exactly what it sounds like. *Prediabetes* is a higher than normal blood glucose level that isn't high enough to be diabetes. One out of three American adults has prediabetes, although many don't know they have it; nine out of ten Americans who have prediabetes are undiagnosed.

Why does prediabetes matter? Well, it turns out that making changes to the foods you eat or exercising more can reduce your risk for diabetes. This is especially true for people with prediabetes. Finding out you have prediabetes can be a wakeup call to make changes to your lifestyle and health.

In one study called the Diabetes Prevention Program, people with prediabetes who lost 5–7 percent of their body weight through changes to diet and exercise reduced their risk of developing diabetes by 58 percent during the 3-year course of the study. This was a landmark study that showed that people at risk for type 2 diabetes can make changes to prevent or delay the disease.

How Is Diabetes Diagnosed?

A healthcare provider can diagnose diabetes by measuring the amount of glucose in your blood using a simple blood test. There are four main tests:

» **A1C test:** The A1C test is also called the hemoglobin A1C, HbA1C, glycated hemoglobin, or glycosylated hemoglobin test. Whew, that's a lot of different names for one test. To keep things simple, we'll refer to it as the A1C test.

The A1C test measures your average blood glucose over 3 months. It's a picture of your blood glucose over time. It actually measures the percentage of hemoglobin (a protein) in your blood that has been *glycated* or attached to glucose over the past three months. You'll hear the number as a percentage such as 7 percent. A1C can be used both to diagnose diabetes and to measure how well you are managing your diabetes if you have it.

For diagnosis, an A1C of 6.5 percent or more means you have diabetes. Prediabetes can be diagnosed with an A1C of 5.7–6.4 percent.

You'll probably hear a lot more about your A1C because it's the test most commonly used to evaluate your diabetes. Your provider will give you an A1C test at every visit or at least three times a year. You can eat or drink what you want before you have an A1C test, so there's no need to fast.

» **Fasting plasma glucose test:** A fasting plasma glucose test can be used to diagnose diabetes. It's also a simple blood test, and it measures your blood glucose as a snapshot in that moment. So, it's different from the A1C, which measures your blood glucose over several months. You can't eat or drink anything besides water for 8 hours before a fasting plasma glucose test.

A reading of 126 mg/dL or above means you have diabetes. Prediabetes can be diagnosed with a fasting plasma glucose of 100–125 mg/dL.

» **Random plasma glucose test:** A random plasma glucose test is another test to diagnose diabetes. Just like it sounds, it can be done "randomly" as a snapshot of your blood glucose. Sometimes healthcare providers do this test if you have other clear signs of diabetes. A reading of 200 mg/dL or above means you have diabetes.

» **Oral glucose tolerance test:** An oral glucose tolerance test can also diagnose diabetes by measuring how well the body uses glucose. You don't eat or drink anything besides water for 8 hours before the test. Upon arrival at the doctor's office, you'll have your blood drawn for a baseline measure. Then you'll drink a liquid with 75 grams of glucose. You'll have your blood drawn 2 hours later. If your reading is 200 mg/dL 2 hours after drinking the liquid, you have diabetes.

Table 1-1 shows the different types of tests used to diagnose diabetes and lists the readings that indicate whether you have diabetes or prediabetes.

TABLE 1-1

Criteria to Diagnose Diabetes

Test	Reading	Diagnosis
A1C	5.7%–6.4%	Prediabetes
	6.5% or above	Diabetes
Fasting plasma glucose	100–125 mg/dL	Prediabetes
	126 mg/dL or above	Diabetes
Random plasma glucose	200 mg/dL or above	Diabetes
Oral glucose tolerance test	200 mg/dL or above two hours after	Diabetes

Understanding Risk Factors

No one knows exactly why some people get diabetes and other people don't get diabetes. There is not a single test that can predict whether you'll develop type 2 diabetes. Instead, type 2 diabetes develops because of a combination of genetic and environmental factors. There isn't just one trigger.

However, there are known risk factors for type 2 diabetes that include your family history, race, ethnicity, and lifestyle. Finding out your risk for diabetes may empower you to make changes such as exercising more or quitting smoking.

Age is a significant risk factor because more people 45 years and older have type 2 diabetes than younger people. Everyone 45 years or older should be tested for type 2 diabetes once they reach 45 years of age and then every 2 years after that.

Family history is another important risk factor. Having a mom or dad, brother, or sister with type 2 diabetes puts you at risk, too. The genes you've inherited are a risk factor, although no one has pinpointed a "diabetes gene."

Your race and ethnicity can also put you at risk for type 2 diabetes. Native Americans, African Americans, Hispanics, Asian Americans, and Pacific Island Americans all have a higher risk of diabetes than non-Hispanic whites. African Americans and Hispanics are over 50 percent more likely to develop diabetes than non-Hispanic whites.

Gestational diabetes is another risk factor that gives moms and their babies a life-time risk of type 2 diabetes. Women with gestational diabetes should be tested for diabetes after they give birth and then every 3 years. Staying active and breast-feeding your baby can help prevent type 2 diabetes later.

High blood pressure, bad cholesterol, and triglycerides also increase your risk for diabetes and heart disease. Smoking or using other tobacco products are contributors, too.

Use the following checklist to determine your risk for developing type 2 diabetes. If you have several risk factors, talk to your doctor about being tested. You can also go to www.diabetes.org/risktest to discover your risk for type 2 diabetes.

>> Getting older, particularly people over 45 years.

>> Being overweight.

>> Having a family history of type 2 diabetes.

>> Race/ethnicity: Native Americans, African Americans, Hispanics, Asian Americans, and Pacific Islanders have a greater risk of type 2 diabetes than non-Hispanic whites.

>> Gestational diabetes.

>> High blood pressure.

>> High "bad" cholesterol and low "good" cholesterol.

>> Not getting much physical activity.

Who Else Has Diabetes?

At the beginning of the chapter, you found out that over 30 million people in the United States have diabetes. In 2015, 1.5 million Americans (18 years old or older) were diagnosed with diabetes.

Americans aren't alone in their struggles against diabetes. About 422 million people had diabetes worldwide in 2014, with people in low- and middle-income countries struggling the most for access to basic care. Worldwide, its prevalence has nearly doubled from 1980 to 2014, according to the World Health Organization.

The statistics around diabetes are stark. And there is much work to be done. Understanding the basics of this disease is an important step in taking action for yourself and for your family and friends, too.

Chapter **2**

Where Do I Begin?

Where do I begin? That's a question many people with diabetes ask themselves. For some people, the question may come up as soon as they're diagnosed with type 2 diabetes. For other people, the question may arise after noticing complications of their diabetes. And still others may face that question as they care for a loved one with diabetes.

It's not easy to know how to start taking care of yourself and managing your diabetes. After all, the diagnosis may have been a total shock. And you may not have a clue about how diabetes will affect your body and your life.

Stay tuned because we're here to help you figure out how to begin taking care of yourself. In this chapter, you discover why it's important to take care of your diabetes on a daily basis and for years to come. You also find out about the basics of managing your diabetes.

REMEMBER

You're the person who will be responsible for making healthy choices each day. You'll make these choices around food, exercise, medications, and even testing your blood glucose. So, let's get started.

Taking Care of Yourself

Making yourself a priority is one of the best steps toward taking care of your diabetes. Yes, *you* are a priority. After all, only you can manage your diabetes. It's not your endocrinologist or your wife or your son who is dealing with diabetes every day. It's you.

Feel better most days

Start taking care of your diabetes so you can feel better most days. Perhaps leading up to your diagnosis of diabetes, you didn't feel so great. You may have gained weight. Or you may have had symptoms of diabetes such as dehydration and blurry vision. Perhaps you were more irritable and out-of-sorts than usual.

In some ways, it may have felt like a relief to discover a cause for these issues. In other ways, it may have felt scary to find out that diabetes was the answer.

The good news is that you can feel great living with type 2 diabetes most days. Not every day is going to be a home run, but most days can be base hits. That's because taking care of yourself and managing your diabetes can positively impact your daily life.

Keeping your blood glucose on target can improve your mood and give you more energy. High blood glucose happens when you have undiagnosed diabetes or when your blood glucose is not on target (see Chapter 1 for more about blood glucose). High blood glucose can make you feel tired, irritable, and thirsty. It may cause you to urinate a lot or blur your vision. Keeping your blood glucose on target with an A1C below 7 percent will reduce the chances of these symptoms.

Two ways to keep your blood glucose on target are to eat healthy foods and exercise regularly. You'll find out more about these two topics in Chapters 11–13.

REMEMBER

Exercise in and of itself is a mood booster. It can reduce stress, lessen symptoms of depression, and release those amazing brain chemicals called *endorphins,* which make you feel good. So even though you may be exercising to help manage your diabetes, you'll have the bonus effect of improving your mood on a daily basis.

Reduce the risk of complications

In the long term, untreated diabetes can really take a toll on your body. Why? It goes back to that issue of high blood glucose we talk about in Chapter 1. With diabetes, glucose gets trapped in the blood because it can't get inside cells to provide energy. When glucose builds up in blood vessels, it creates a recipe for disaster.

High blood glucose damages blood vessels. People with diabetes also have an increased risk of high blood pressure, which can make things worse; blood vessels can't pump enough blood or nutrients to all the parts of your body, and they can die or become clogged.

Blood vessels are everywhere in your body. They're in your heart, eyes, toes, penis or vagina, intestines, and brain. High blood glucose affects all these blood vessels. It is an equal-opportunity blood vessel destroyer.

Blood vessel problems fall into two categories:

>> **Microvascular:** Your small blood vessels. Complications can include the following:

- **Damage to small blood vessels in your eyes:** This can lead to ruptures and unhealthy regrowth, which can cause vision impairment or blindness.

- **Damage to small blood vessels in your kidneys:** This affects their ability to filter. And overworked vessels can lead to kidney failure.

- **Damage to capillaries throughout your body:** This could affect how quickly wounds heal.

>> **Macrovascular:** Your large blood vessels. Complications can include the following:

- **Damage to the large blood vessels in your heart:** This can lead to heart attacks, heart failure, and death.

- **Damage to large blood vessels in your brain:** This can cause strokes and death.

- **Damage to large blood vessels in your legs:** This causes peripheral artery disease, a painful condition that makes moving painful.

Now it's easy to understand why diabetes affects so many parts of your body. Uncontrolled blood glucose increases your risk of heart disease, stroke, kidney failure, blindness, nerve loss, and even amputation. Find out more about complications and how to prevent them in Chapter 8.

Keeping your blood vessels healthy is one of the holy grails of managing your diabetes. It may not sound exciting: "I took a bike ride today and improved my blood vessels." But it's why it's important to take care of yourself and manage your blood glucose and diabetes.

TECHNICAL
STUFF

The UK Prospective Diabetes Study showed that improving blood glucose and/or blood pressure reduced complications of type 2 diabetes. In this 20-year landmark study, scientists learned that complications were not inevitable for people with type 2 diabetes.

Healthy pregnancy, healthy baby

Taking care of your diabetes is important if you're thinking about becoming pregnant. Try to get your blood glucose under control *before* you become pregnant and avoid an unplanned pregnancy if you have type 2 diabetes.

Before you become pregnant, try to lose weight if you need to, and get active. Make sure your A1C is within your target range. Talk to your doctor about your plans and make sure you've had a complete checkup, including a dilated eye exam. Eye disease can progress rapidly during pregnancy for some women. All these steps will set you up for success once you conceive.

WARNING

High blood glucose can harm your baby during the first few weeks after conception, even if you don't know you're pregnant yet. It can cause birth defects in the developing baby such as heart or brain problems.

During your pregnancy, you may need to take medications such as insulin to manage your blood glucose. You may also need to adjust the foods you eat. Your hormone levels change during pregnancy, and they can affect your blood glucose, so you may need to revamp your regimen. Keeping your blood glucose under control will help you prevent complications such as *preeclampsia* (involving high blood pressure) or having a large baby with injuries during birth.

Taking care of your blood glucose during your pregnancy (and before) will help keep you and your baby healthy. See Chapter 9 for more details about diabetes and pregnancy.

Managing Your Diabetes

You may have heard the terms *diabetes self-management plan* or *diabetes care plan*. Both of these terms refer to how you take care of or manage your diabetes. Your plan takes into account your big-picture goals and your nitty-gritty choices each day.

On the one hand, diabetes management is not a small endeavor. You're the person most responsible for taking care of your diabetes 24 hours a day, 7 days a week, 365 days a year. It's not your diabetes educator or endocrinologist or even your spouse who will carry the torch. It's you, the person with diabetes.

On the other hand, it's a well-trodden road. Many, many people just like you are learning to test their blood glucose, take new medications, and change the way they eat and exercise. There are millions of people in towns and cities across the United States managing their diabetes with successes and struggles. You can find them in your community hospital's diabetes support group, and you can find them online on the American Diabetes Association's message boards. You're not alone — and there's much to learn from your healthcare team and others with type 2 diabetes.

This book walks you through the basics of managing your diabetes, chapter by chapter and step by step. In the following sections, we give you an overview about putting together a healthcare team, taking medications, eating healthy foods, getting active, and finding support.

Assembling a healthcare team

One of the first steps you'll take in managing your diabetes is to put together your healthcare team. At first, you may start with your diabetes care provider, who may be your family physician or nurse practitioner or an endocrinologist. You'll probably see a *certified diabetes educator* (CDE), who is specially trained to help people manage their diabetes. These professionals will monitor your diabetes and any related complications, but also help you set goals and troubleshoot problems as they arise.

Other specialists you may see include dietitians, ophthalmologists, podiatrists, dermatologists, and others. Read more about your healthcare team and what to expect during checkups in Chapters 3 and 4.

Taking medications

You may be prescribed a medication, such as metformin, as soon as you're diagnosed with diabetes. Or you may take a combination of medications or insulin injections. Taking your prescribed medications is an essential piece of managing your type 2 diabetes. It is a cornerstone of your care — and it's important to do it at the correct times each day or each week.

REMEMBER

Switching a medication, adding a medication, or taking insulin is a normal part of having diabetes. Your diabetes will change over time, and your medication needs may change, too. Find out more about the different types of diabetes medications and how they work in Chapter 6.

Checking blood glucose

Your healthcare provider will test your blood glucose using the A1C test during your checkups. As we explain in Chapter 1, an A1C test is a measure of your blood glucose over the previous three months. It gauges how well your medications work or whether you need to change your meals or physical activity.

You may also be asked to check your blood glucose on your own using a meter. You'll prick your skin using a lancet to draw a drop of blood, press a test strip onto the blood, and then get a reading on your meter. We walk you through all these steps in Chapter 7.

REMEMBER

Checking your blood glucose will help you see how different things like food, exercise, and medications affect your blood glucose. It's a snapshot of your diabetes that can help you make informed decisions like choosing a smaller meal at lunchtime or walking an extra 20 minutes in the evening when you get home from work.

Eating healthy and staying active

Learning about wholesome, nutritious foods and how to incorporate them into meals is a critical part of managing your diabetes. You may not have thought much about the nutritional benefits of certain foods before you were diagnosed with type 2 diabetes. After all, we all eat foods because they taste good. That's the fun part!

You don't have to give up your favorite foods because you have diabetes. Instead, you may need to eat them in smaller portions or prepare them differently to reduce calories. You may also add a few new foods packed with nutritional punch like salmon, beets, and olive oil.

Exercising also helps manage your diabetes by moving glucose out of the bloodstream and making your cells more sensitive to insulin. It boosts your mood and distracts you from everyday worries. Read all about food and physical activity in Chapters 11–13.

Finding support

Perhaps it sounds touchy-feely, but finding support is another important part of managing your diabetes. Support can mean so many different things — from chatting with online buddies on a message board to attending a diabetes education class.

At some point, you may experience the very real feelings associated with diabetes distress, including fatigue, annoyance, and just plain burnout. Or you may experience more intense emotions of depression and/or an anxiety disorder.

TIP

Talk to your healthcare provider about your feelings and concerns and seek support from a mental health professional or others with type 2 diabetes. Get more tips for dealing with stress and getting in touch with yourself in Chapter 14.

2

Your Healthcare Team and Medications

Chapter 3

Putting Together Your Healthcare Team

Building a trusted group of physicians, nurses, and specialists is an important part of your diabetes care. It may be helpful to think of this group as a team because they'll be working together to ensure that you have the best access to care and tools for managing your diabetes.

You're in charge of the team, in terms of assembling these healthcare providers and making sure they communicate with one another. Your team members may practice together as part of a center that specializes in diabetes care, which makes this coordination more straightforward. Or your diabetes care provider may recommend that you see other specialists, and in that case, you'll be responsible for making those appointments and making sure those people share your health records.

You may not have thought of healthcare as a team effort, but it's actually a good way to think about taking care of your body. After all, diabetes affects every part of your body from your mind to your stomach to your toes. Consider the option to consult with physicians and nurses with various experience and expertise.

In this chapter, we tell you about the central players on your team, such as your primary care provider, endocrinologist, nurse practitioner, or certified diabetes educator. You also find out about other specialists such as dietitians, eye doctors, podiatrists, pharmacists, dentists, dermatologists, and exercise physiologists. Along the way, we give you tips on how to select these providers and what to expect when you visit their offices.

TIP

Don't be overwhelmed by assembling your team all at once. At the beginning, you may simply start by seeing your diabetes care provider and a certified diabetes educator. You may already have some members of your team onboard such as a dentist and pharmacist. And you'll build the rest of your team as your healthcare needs change over time.

Starting with a Diabetes Care Provider

Your diabetes care provider is your go-to person. A diabetes care provider might be your primary care provider whom you've known for years and years. It could be a family practitioner, internist, or nurse practitioner, and that provider may have been the person who first diagnosed you with type 2 diabetes.

You may also choose to see an *endocrinologist,* a physician trained to treat people with hormone imbalances including diabetes. You may find this training and expertise helpful in managing your diabetes.

Don't worry, you don't have to say goodbye to your primary care provider if you see an endocrinologist. Instead, you may see an endocrinologist in addition to your primary care provider, who will help you manage any other health concerns.

A diabetes care provider will give you a yearly physical exam and an A1C test every 3–6 months. You find out more specifics about those checkups in the next chapter.

TIP

You can find nurse practitioners in primary and specialty care. A nurse practitioner may be at the center of your diabetes care team. Nurse practitioners can make diagnoses, prescribe medications, order lab tests, and develop a diabetes management plan. They have advanced clinical training beyond a registered nurse (RN) so look out for the credentials NP. Physician assistants (PAs) can be primary care providers. They can diagnose and treat patients and prescribe medicines. Their roles vary depending on the healthcare setting, their experience, and their specialty. They can have specialized training in treating people with diabetes.

Choosing the right provider for you

If you decide to find a clinician who specializes in diabetes care instead of using your primary care provider, put some time and effort into choosing someone who is a good fit for you. After all, you'll likely be seeing this person a couple of times a year for the rest of your life.

Do your homework by looking into their education, medical certification, experience, and insurance acceptance. Many providers and offices have websites where you can find out these details beforehand. For example, the office website might have a short bio and photograph of providers.

Here are some questions to ask about the physician's education and experience:

>> Where did the provider go to medical school?

>> Is the provider board certified in endocrinology or internal medicine?

>> Does the provider have professional memberships in associations such as the American Diabetes Association or the American Association of Clinical Endocrinologists?

>> Does the provider see a lot of people with diabetes? Type 1 or type 2?

The logistics of care, philosophy, and demeanor of a potential provider are other things to mull over. For example, is it easy to schedule a same-day appointment with the provider in case of an emergency? How can you get in touch when you have questions about managing your blood glucose?

You may need to schedule an interview with the provider to get answers to these questions, or you may be able to ask these questions during your first visit. When you first call the office, ask whether the office has a new patient packet or whether you'll have the opportunity to ask these types of questions. A physician may charge an interview fee for these types of visits.

Don't be afraid to make a list of questions ahead of time and bring them with you. Write down the answers so you remember them later. Here's a list of questions to get you started:

>> How often should I expect to see you? What exams or tests are done in those visits?

>> Who covers for you on your days off?

>> How does your office handle emergencies, and whom can I expect to talk to?

>> Can I schedule a same-day appointment for urgent matters?

>> Do you work with a certified diabetes educator, dietitian, or other specialists to coordinate my diabetes care?

>> How do you view the patient and provider relationship?

>> Can I call or email with questions? How do you prefer to communicate?

>> How would you describe your communication style?

After your first visit, take time to reflect on the experience. If you felt comfortable talking to the provider, that's a good sign. Try to find a provider with whom you feel at ease talking about your feelings and concerns. That provider should also be willing to work with you toward your individual goals. Part of that willingness is an ability to listen.

REMEMBER

Your endocrinologist or primary care provider may have other staff that you interact with regularly such as nurses, nurse practitioners, and physician assistants (PAs). These people are also part of your healthcare team. And they may have more availability than your regular physician. Ask the office whether you'll contact these providers regularly, using a nurse's on-call hot line for example.

TIP

Recommendations from friends and family are great ways to find a trusted diabetes care provider. If you know someone with diabetes, ask him whether he likes his provider and why. Other physicians can also be good sources of information. If you love your optometrist, ask her whether she would recommend an endocrinologist in the area.

Considering insurance coverage

As you're selecting a diabetes care provider, keep a few things in mind such as health insurance coverage and convenience.

Make sure your provider is covered under your health insurance plan by talking to someone at the phone number listed on your health insurance card. You can also call your health insurance company or go online for a listing of covered endocrinologists or other specialists in your area.

Consider the location of the provider's office and how convenient it will be to get to appointments two or more times a year. For example, if the nearest endocrinologist is more than an hour a way, you may opt to see a primary care provider who specializes in diabetes instead.

After you've chosen a diabetes care provider, ask him or her the following questions:

» Do you accept my health insurance? (Even if you confirmed with your health insurance company that it works with your doctor, it doesn't hurt to confirm that with the doctor's office.)

» Are you a provider in my PPO or HMO plan?

» If I need a referral to see a specialist, do you have colleagues who participate under my health insurance plan?

Adding a Certified Diabetes Educator

A *certified diabetes educator* (CDE) is the other key player on your healthcare team. In fact, a diabetes educator may be the first person to really tell you about diabetes: what it is and how you can manage it daily.

A CDE is your go-to person for education and management questions. Her goal is to make managing your diabetes easier in your everyday life. For example, a CDE can help you develop a plan to eat healthful foods, get physically active, and take your medications. Her goal is to get to know you, answer questions, and help you troubleshoot problems. After all, you're the one taking care of your diabetes most of the time: A CDE is the health professional whose job it is to help you do that effectively.

A diabetes educator can be a registered nurse, nurse practitioner, registered dietitian, pharmacist, podiatrist, or psychologist with training to educate and care for people with diabetes. Physicians and physician assistants can also be diabetes educators. A CDE's role on your healthcare team depends on her specialty and the office setting or hospital where she practices.

A CDE has received credentials from the National Certification Board for Diabetes Educators by passing an exam and logging a certain number of hours caring for people with diabetes. Look for the letters CDE in the person's credentials when choosing a diabetes educator.

When you're first diagnosed with diabetes, your provider will likely refer you to a CDE or a diabetes education class taught by one. (Find out more about diabetes education classes in Chapter 5.)

Visit a CDE when you're first diagnosed with diabetes, as well as during yearly visits. You can also see a CDE if you have changes to your medications, eating or exercise goals, or other questions about how to tweak your diabetes management plan.

Seeing Other Specialists

Your healthcare team is primarily made up of your diabetes care provider and a CDE. Other specialists can help round out your care by providing specific expertise. You may see a dietitian, ophthalmologist or optometrist, pharmacist, and dentist. An exercise physiologist or trainer, podiatrist, dermatologist, and mental health specialist are other helpful experts.

TIP

Make sure your diabetes care provider has the names, phone numbers, and fax numbers of these other specialists. Ideally, you can share your health records electronically or by fax or email with all your doctors. One of the most important records to share is your medication record. Because medications can have interactions and adverse effects, it's important that each one of your doctors (even your dentist) knows the medications you're currently taking.

Dietitian: Helping you mind your meals

A dietitian is your best bet for getting the latest info on healthy eating. Dietitians are experts in food and nutrition. You may see a dietitian when you're first diagnosed with diabetes and then for yearly visits afterward. A dietitian is a great person to bounce ideas around with when you're having trouble reaching your blood glucose targets.

Developing a plan for healthy meals is one of the core roles of a dietitian. You can work with a dietitian to incorporate foods that you enjoy and that are part of your culture and traditions. It's important to eat foods you love because otherwise it's extremely hard to follow a plan. If you're constantly denying yourself foods that you crave, you're more likely to forgo healthy choices altogether. Instead, find ways to substitute and incorporate pleasurable foods like pizza or buttered popcorn at the movies.

A dietitian should also take into account your lifestyle, health, and physical activity. For example, if you work long hours, you may need to plan ahead for easy snacks and workweek meals so you can make healthy choices when you're short on time. A dietitian can also take into account your health goals such as losing weight, reducing sodium, or cutting back on sugar.

Sometimes people never see a dietitian even though they've lived with diabetes for years. Don't let this happen to you. What you eat is critical when you have type 2 diabetes, so seek out the best advice and expertise with a dietitian.

Ask your diabetes care provider or CDE for a referral to a dietitian. Sometimes your diabetes educator will be a dietitian as well. The Academy of Nutrition and Dietetics has information about types of dietitians and how to find them in your community; for more information, visit www.eatright.org.

A registered dietitian (RD) or a registered dietitian nutritionist (RDN) is a health professional who advises people about meal planning, nutrition, and weight control. They are accredited by the Academy of Nutrition and Dietetics, so look for the letters *RD* or *RDN* after their names.

Individual states also license dietitians, so you may see the letters *LD* after a dietitian's name, which stands for *licensed dietitian*.

TIP

You don't necessarily have to pay out-of-pocket to see a dietitian. In fact, some health insurance plans cover appointments with dietitians because they are considered medical nutrition therapy. Call your health insurance provider to see whether you're covered, and ask whether you'll need a prescription and whether to see specific dietitians that participate in your insurance plan.

Medicare Part B covers medical nutrition therapy and related services for people with diabetes, which could include an initial nutrition and lifestyle assessment, one-on-one nutritional counseling, and follow-up visits. Get a referral from your provider for medical nutrition therapy. For more information, visit www.medicare.gov. In some states, Medicaid may also cover visits with a dietitian. See Chapter 11 for more tips on reimbursement.

Ophthalmologist or optometrist: Keeping an eye on your eyes

An eye specialist such as an ophthalmologist or optometrist should be part of your healthcare team. An ophthalmologist is a doctor of medicine (MD) who specializes in eye care and eye diseases; an optometrist is an eye doctor with a doctor of optometry degree (OD) who diagnoses vision changes and disease and does sight testing and correction.

TIP

Have a comprehensive, dilated eye exam by an ophthalmologist or optometrist when you're first diagnosed with diabetes. After that, you should get an exam every 1–2 years, depending on your sight and diabetes care.

As a person with diabetes, your eyes are particularly vulnerable to vision changes and damage. That's because the blood vessels in your eyes can rupture and swell over time. Diabetic eye disease is the number one cause of blindness among working-age adults in the United States.

The great news is that you can prevent or delay blindness (from diabetic retinopathy) with early detection and treatment. The key to early detection is making an appointment with an ophthalmologist or optometrist yearly for an exam. During a dilated eye exam, an eye specialist can diagnose damage in your eyes even though you may not notice any vision problems on your own. Don't wait until you notice vision changes to see an ophthalmologist or optometrist!

REMEMBER

Seeing an ophthalmologist or optometrist is especially important for women with preexisting diabetes who become pregnant because eye disease can progress rapidly during pregnancy.

Pharmacist: Filling you in on medication details

You may think of your pharmacist as just that person behind the counter who fills and refills your prescriptions. Your pharmacist is that and much more. She is an expert on medications: dosage, uses, and how the drugs interact. A pharmacist is a key member of your healthcare team. If you have diabetes, you're probably not just taking one medication, but perhaps a pill for blood glucose, a pill for high blood pressure, and maybe even another pill for cholesterol. The interaction of these medications can impact your body.

Pharmacists receive a PharmD degree and also licensure in the state where they practice pharmacy.

A pharmacist tells you how often and how much to take of a medication and its potential side effects. If you have a new prescription, ask your pharmacist how it will affect your current medications. Take the opportunity to review all your medications and pinpoint any adverse reactions or symptoms to look out for after you're home.

TIP

Consider keeping all your prescriptions at one pharmacy or consolidating them so your pharmacist knows all your medications. Your pharmacist should have an up-to-date profile on your medical history, allergies, and medications.

A pharmacist is also a great source of information for over-the-counter medications such as cold relievers and upset stomach remedies. Tell your pharmacist about your symptoms, and ask her to recommend a safe and effective treatment.

TIP

If you have trouble keeping track of or remembering to take your medication, ask your pharmacist for help. Your pharmacist may be able to offer specific tips or tools for taking medications daily.

Dentist and dental hygienist: Keeping your mouth in tip-top shape

Good oral care is a top priority for people with diabetes because they may be more susceptible to mouth and gum infections. Elevated blood glucose can encourage infections and can hamper the healing process. The best way to prevent these infections is to brush twice a day and floss. It's good for your mouth — and your breath will thank you, too.

The other way to take care of your teeth, mouth, and gums is to visit a dentist every 6 months for a cleaning. Tell your dentist that you have diabetes and write it down on the paperwork when you check in for your appointment. Make sure to tell your dentist or hygienist about any problems you're experiencing such as dry mouth, bleeding or sensitive gums, or persistent bad breath or bad taste in your mouth.

Exercise physiologist: Focusing on your fitness

Exercise physiologists are health professionals who help you develop a fitness program. They work directly with you to assess your current health — and come up with an exercise plan that fits your goals.

Your diabetes care provider may refer you to an exercise physiologist if you have certain complications like heart or lung problems. An exercise physiologist may have you do stress or fitness tests to evaluate your health and pinpoint concerns. One of the things an exercise physiologist can help you do is develop a personalized plan for exercise.

Exercise physiologists typically have a bachelor's degree, and sometimes a master's degree as well. The American Society of Exercise Physiologists and the American College of Sports Medicine both offer certification programs for exercise physiologists.

TIP

Exercise physiologists are different from personal trainers or fitness instructors. Personal trainers or fitness instructors are primarily focused on helping to instruct or motivate people about exercise. You don't necessarily need a degree to be a personal trainer or instructor, and there are a number of organizations that offer certification for these positions. You can find personal trainers at your local gym or in your community, and they can be great sources of inspiration and education on getting active. Just as with hiring anyone, ask for recommendations from family and friends and look for people with experience helping people with type 2 diabetes.

Podiatrist: Standing up for your feet

Podiatrists are doctors with specialized training to care for and treat foot problems. Podiatrists take care of corns, calluses, and foot sores to prevent more serious infections. A podiatrist can show you how to correctly trim your toenails and take care of your feet daily. They can prescribe and fit you for specialized shoes to make walking and exercising more comfortable.

You may need a podiatrist on your healthcare team because people with diabetes often have poor circulation to their feet and nerve damage. This can make it difficult to feel cuts and sores, so you may not even know you have an infection until it's gotten much worse.

Even though you'll be doing tasks at home to keep your feet healthy, such as checking them daily for infections or sores (see Chapter 8), problems may arise that require the care of a specialist.

WARNING

Don't ignore or try to treat foot problems on your own. Call your diabetes care provider or podiatrist if you have

>> Changes in feeling such as pain, tingling, numbness, or burning

>> A puncture wound from stepping on a nail or thorn

>> An open sore (called an *ulcer*)

>> A cut or sore that isn't healing

>> An infection in a cut or blister

>> A red, tender toe

Also, your diabetes care provider will check out your feet during a physical exam. It's part of your routine evaluation, so take off those socks and shoes when you walk in the room for your appointment. That way, you'll both remember to check your feet and talk about any problems or pain.

You can ask for a referral to a podiatrist if you have more severe foot problems that your diabetes care provider doesn't feel comfortable treating.

Podiatrists receive a doctor of podiatric medicine (DPM) from a college of podiatry. They gain expertise by doing residence training in podiatry and train to perform surgery and prescribe medication for your feet.

Dermatologist: Helping your skin stay healthy

If you're having issues with your skin, a dermatologist can help. Dermatologists are medical doctors (MDs) with a specialty in diagnosing and treating skin disorders. People with diabetes may have problems with their skin because high blood glucose can cause dehydration and dry or moist skin can cause skin infections. Ask for a referral to a dermatologist if you have skin problems. They can tell you how to take care of your skin to prevent dryness and infections, as well as prescribe medications to treat these issues.

Mental health specialist: Minding your thoughts and emotions

Your mind and emotions are just as important as your physical health. In fact, the two are closely entwined. Living with a chronic condition such as diabetes can be exhausting and annoying. And it can also lead to conditions such as diabetes burnout, depression, and anxiety. Don't be afraid to bring these issues up, even if your provider doesn't specifically ask about your mental health. (See more about emotions and coping in Chapter 14.)

Mental health specialists are trained to help you cope with these sometimes overwhelming thoughts and emotions. There are a wide range of specialists, so consider your needs and the cost. Here's an overview of the different types of mental health specialists:

>> A **psychiatrist** is a medical doctor (MD) who can prescribe medications or other treatments and offer therapy. You may try to find a psychiatrist with experience treating people with diabetes.

>> A **clinical psychologist** has a master's or doctoral degree in psychology and training to help people with depression, anxiety, or other problems. A psychologist may specialize in individual, group, or family psychology. They receive a license to practice from their state.

» A **marriage or family therapist** has a master's or doctoral degree in mental health and training in therapy for married couples and families going through stressful periods.

» A **social worker** has a master's degree in social work (MSW) and works across a broad range of categories such as coping with workplace stresses, family and marital problems, and identifying resources in the community for those who need financial, educational, or medical help.

Some health plans cover mental healthcare, while many others don't offer this coverage. Ask your diabetes care provider for a referral or recommendation to a mental health professional.

REMEMBER

You may need to see a kidney doctor, called a *nephrologist*, if your diabetes care provider recommends it. People with diabetes are more likely to have problems with their kidneys because high blood glucose can damage blood vessels in these organs.

Chapter **4**

Your Checkups

C heckups with your diabetes care provider are wonderful opportunities to discuss your goals and measure your progress in managing your diabetes. They're also critical appointments to evaluate your blood glucose and assess any other problems that may have arisen recently.

In this chapter, we tell you what to expect during office visits and what to bring with you. You also find out about the types of physical exams and lab tests typical for people with type 2 diabetes. And don't forget vaccines; you'll find out about one-time and yearly vaccinations to keep you healthy throughout the seasons. Good communication is another important skill to master with your healthcare provider, so we also offer tips on the best ways to talk to your provider and make sure your concerns are heard.

What to Expect in a Checkup

There is a lot to do at your visit with your diabetes care provider. Try to prepare and plan ahead so your visit goes smoothly. Here, we tell you what to expect so you can get the most out of your appointment, including the skinny on blood glucose, blood pressure, and cholesterol. You also find out what to ask about medications and your plan for meals and physical activity.

Blood glucose roundup

During your first visit with your diabetes care provider, you'll come up with a plan for managing your diabetes. Work with your provider to determine clear goals for your blood glucose, including if and when to check it with a blood glucose meter on your own. Your provider may say you don't need to check it at all if you're not taking medications, or you may need to check it several times a day if you take insulin. Ask your provider what she recommends.

Part of this discussion is creating a plan for your daily blood glucose targets. For example, many people with diabetes shoot for a fasting blood glucose of 80–130 mg/dL. Your fasting blood glucose is normally the test that you do in the morning before you eat anything. Another common target is 2 hours after a meal of less than 180 mg/dL.

When you check your blood glucose levels, the numbers will be stored in your blood glucose meter. (See more about meters and how to check your blood glucose in Chapter 7.) Your provider may recommend that you write these numbers down in a separate paper logbook or record them in an app or spreadsheet. This can help you see trends in your blood glucose, especially in reaction to changes of medications, foods, or physical activity.

The A1C test is another way to measure your blood glucose over time; your provider does this simple blood test in the office. It's usually done two or more times a year, depending on your health and blood glucose control.

A1C is a measure of your average blood glucose over 3 months, so this number is helpful for both you and your provider to measure how your overall diabetes plan is working. Many people with type 2 diabetes have an A1C goal of less than 7 percent. However, you and your provider may decide that you want a more or less stringent goal for your A1C. Ask your provider to tell you your A1C level and write it down so you remember it later. Ask your provider whether your A1C is on target; if it's not, ask how you can improve it. A1C is used to evaluate key points in your blood glucose management including your medication, food choices, weight, and physical activity. Don't be shy about knowing this number and whether it's in the ideal range.

TIP

Your provider may also give your A1C result as eAG or estimated average glucose. This unit of measurement is similar to the units given during readings from the blood glucose meter that you use on your own. A1C is a percentage; eAG is given in mg/dL.

REMEMBER

Many people with diabetes try for an A1C of 7 percent or less, so ask your provider if this number is right for you.

Weight matters

You'll step on the scale during each visit to see whether you've lost or gained weight. Losing or maintaining weight can help you keep your blood glucose in your target range, so it's an important measurement for anyone with type 2 diabetes.

Your height will also be recorded. The ratio of your height and weight is called *body mass index* (BMI), and it's used to determine whether you're underweight, normal, overweight, or obese. A BMI of 25 mg/k² (23 mg/k² for Asian Americans) or higher could mean that you need to lose weight, and a BMI of 27 mg/k² or higher, coupled with your diabetes, could mean you're a candidate for weight-loss medications. If you have type 2 diabetes and a BMI of 35 mg/k² or higher, you may consider bariatric surgery. See more about bariatric surgery in Chapter 6.

Fluctuations in weight — up or down — may also mean you need to adjust your medications, meals, or physical activity.

Setting goals for food and exercise

Work with your provider to come up with a plan for healthy eating and more physical activity. This includes both a discussion of daily food goals and weekly exercise goals. See more about both in Chapters 12 and 13.

Ask whether to plan for a certain number of calories or carbohydrates per day. Ask whether to target specific goals for limiting sodium or sugar. Write these goals down so you can refer to them later. Bring up any concerns you're having at mealtimes or difficulties you're having with eating or avoiding certain foods. Your provider may recommend that you see a certified diabetes educator (CDE) or dietitian to work on a more detailed plan.

Exercise is another topic of discussion during your checkup. Ask how long and how often to exercise every week. Write the plan down so you can refer to it later. Then keep track of your physical activity so you can talk about it with your provider at your next visit.

TIP

Tell your provider if you're having trouble getting started or keeping up with regular physical activity. Pain, soreness, and fatigue are common symptoms that get in the way of being active, so tell your provider if you're experiencing these issues so you can find treatments or alternative exercises.

Medication roundup

You can also expect to run through your medications and how they're working with your provider. Your provider will use your A1C test and perhaps your blood glucose readings to evaluate how well your medications are working to manage your blood glucose.

Tell your provider about any new medications or supplements you may have started taking since your last appointment. It's important for your provider to have the most up-to-date list of your current medications and doses. If you're seeing a new provider, consider putting all the medications from your medicine cabinet into a brown bag and taking it with you to the appointment. That way, you won't forget the name and doses of any medications.

TIP

If you're experiencing new symptoms or side effects, tell your provider. They may be linked to a medication and its dosage. Or that medication could be interacting with another medication. Your provider's job is to troubleshoot these issues, so don't be afraid to bring up any concerns.

Ask your doctor about the dose and timing of each medication you're taking, especially if he prescribes a new one. Some medications may be taken with food, so you need to know these details. See Chapter 6 for more about medications.

Targets for blood pressure and cholesterol

Your blood pressure and cholesterol are also closely linked to your diabetes and overall health. People with diabetes are at risk for damage to blood vessels in their heart, eyes, kidneys, feet, and other parts of their body. This can lead to all kinds of problems such as heart attacks, blindness, kidney failure, and amputation.

High blood pressure and bad cholesterol can both exacerbate blood vessel damage, so the goal is to keep these numbers low. Good cholesterol keeps blood vessels healthy. Eating wholesome nutritious foods, losing or maintaining a healthy weight, exercising, and taking medications can all reduce blood pressure and bad cholesterol and raise good cholesterol.

You'll have your blood pressure taken at each checkup. Most people with diabetes have a goal of less than 140 mmHg systolic blood pressure and less than 90 mmHg diastolic blood pressure. If your blood pressure is higher than this, your provider may recommend changes to your foods, exercise, or new medications. Reducing salt, quitting smoking, and eating whole-grain foods can lower blood pressure.

You're not alone if you have high blood pressure. One in three Americans has high blood pressure, and two in three people with diabetes have high blood pressure or take medications to lower it. Keeping an eye on blood pressure is a good idea because high blood pressure increases the risk of stroke and heart disease — problems that people with diabetes already have a higher risk for.

Peripheral arterial disease (PAD) occurs when arteries in your legs narrow and become blocked; it can cause pain in your legs, hips, and other parts of the body. Tell your provider if you have these symptoms so she can test for PAD using a simple test that measures blood pressure at your arm and ankle. It's called the ankle/brachial index. (See Chapter 8 for more about PAD.)

You'll have a blood test for your cholesterol when you're first diagnosed with diabetes, and then every 5 years or more frequently depending on your doctor's recommendation. You can lower your bad cholesterol and boost your good cholesterol by reducing animal fats and eating plant fats like avocados, olive oil, and legumes. You can also take medications such as statins to lower your bad cholesterol.

Cholesterol is a type of blood fat, and it can clog arteries and lead to heart disease, stroke, and other blood vessel problems. Cholesterol is divided into two types:

>> **Low-density lipoprotein (LDL) cholesterol** is called "bad" cholesterol because it can build up in your arteries. The lower your LDL cholesterol, the better.

>> **High-density lipoprotein (HDL) cholesterol** is called "good" cholesterol because it removes cholesterol from the body. In this case, the higher, the better.

Triglycerides are another blood fat that increases your risk of heart disease and stroke. Again, the lower, the better.

Kidney tests

Kidneys are the underappreciated workhorses of our bodies, filtering out toxins through our urine and returning necessary nutrients to our bodies. However, this amazing filtration system can deteriorate when blood vessels in your kidneys narrow and clog. This can lead to kidney disease and, in some cases, kidney failure.

Two simple tests measure your kidney function, and they both have funky names. Serum creatinine/eGFR is a blood test, and urine albumin-to-creatinine ratio is a urine test. Get both tests yearly if you have type 2 diabetes.

Foot check

Take off your socks and shoes when you enter the exam room so both you and your provider remember to do a foot check. Your provider should carefully examine your feet for any sores, cuts, or other visible problems. He should also test for signs of nerve damage by examining your reflexes and asking you about pain or loss of sensation. Tell your physician about any problems you've experienced with your feet or nail care. Your diabetes care provider or podiatrist should do a foot evaluation every year or more frequently if you have foot issues.

Vaccinations

Get a flu shot each year to try to prevent influenza, which can be more severe for people over 65 years of age or those with an underlying condition like diabetes. Ask about vaccinations against pneumococcal pneumonia, which is a common complication of the flu and can cause dangerous infections.

The American Diabetes Association also recommends that people with diabetes 19–59 years old have the hepatitis B vaccine because they are at higher risk for this infection. Get the Tdap (whooping cough, diphtheria, tetanus), Zoster (shingles) if 60 years of age or older, Varicella (chicken pox), and MMR (measles, mumps, rubella) vaccines.

You can find a vaccination list schedule for adults and children at the website of the Centers for Disease Control and Prevention (www.cdc.gov/vaccines/schedules).

Here's a handy list you can refer to in order to make sure you're getting the right vaccinations to keep you healthy:

>> **Flu vaccine:** A shot once a year, ideally in the fall. Doctor's offices and pharmacies carry the flu vaccine, which is reformulated each year to combat the most common strains expected that year.

>> **Pneumococcal pneumonia:** The two types of pneumococcal pneumonia vaccines are PCV13 and PPSV23. Vaccination with PCV13 is recommended for children before age 2 years. People with diabetes ages 2–64 years should also receive PPSV23. For all adults 65 years or older, regardless of vaccination history, an additional PPSV23 vaccination is necessary.

>> **Hepatitis B:** A series of three vaccines for adults with diabetes ages 19–59 years (may be considered in people 60 years and older). Given as a 3-dose series.

>> **Tdap:** For whooping cough, diphtheria, and tetanus. All adults who did not get Tdap during adolescence should get one dose. A Tdap booster should be given every 10 years.

>> **Zoster:** For shingles if you're 60 or older. It's a one-time dose.

>> **Varicella:** To prevent chicken pox. If never received as a child, 1–2 doses, with timing determined by the doctor.

>> **MMR:** To prevent measles, mumps, and rubella. If never received as a child, ask your provider about her recommendation.

Extra time for questions and concerns

It may seem like all of the above is a lot to cover in one checkup. And it is. But all these tests and discussions are important components of your diabetes care.

TIP

Make time for any questions or concerns at the beginning or end of your checkup. It may be helpful for you to write down your questions ahead of time and bring them with you. And it can be a good idea to start the appointment by telling your provider that you have questions and asking her about an ideal time to discuss them during the checkup.

Making Time for a Yearly Eye Exam

Have a comprehensive eye exam every 1–2 years to check for signs of damage or disease. An optometrist or ophthalmologist does this exam in his office, which is usually separate from your diabetes care provider. However, some primary care offices may have technicians or specialists available to do these eye exams.

As part of the exam, the optometrist or ophthalmologist will dilate your eyes with drops and then use a magnifying glass to look at the retina for signs of damage. Sometimes the blood vessels rupture and leak, causing damage. Oftentimes, you won't have symptoms such as trouble seeing during the early stages of eye disease. That's why it's so important to see an eye specialist every year to detect any damage to your eyes. If your eye exam is completely normal, your eye specialist may recommend an exam every other year.

REMEMBER

Your eyes are so important! Don't neglect this exam even though it may be a chore to schedule or to get there each year. Diabetic eye disease is the leading cause of blindness in American adults. Yet, it can be treated very successfully with injections or lasers if detected early.

Your Checkup Schedule in a Nutshell

Each year, you'll get a series of physical exams and lab tests for your diabetes. We've covered them in detail earlier in this chapter, but we'll also outline them here in checklist form.

Physical exams and appointments

❑ Weight and height measurements for calculating BMI (every visit)

❑ Blood pressure measurement (every visit)

❑ Foot check with diabetes care provider (every visit) or podiatrist (once a year or more often if you have problems)

❑ Setting goals for food and exercise with diabetes care provider, nurse, physician assistant, or CDE (once a year or more often)

❑ Discussion of medications, old and new, as well as refills of prescriptions (every visit)

❑ Comprehensive dilated eye exam by optometrist or ophthalmologist (once a year; every other year if your eye specialist recommends)

❑ Teeth cleaning (every 6 months) and mouth exam (once a year) by dental hygienist and dentist, as a general rule

❑ Ankle-brachial index test if you have signs of PAD (as needed)

Lab tests

❑ A1C test, by diabetes care provider (blood test/2–4 times a year)

❑ Cholesterol measurements for LDL and HDL cholesterol, and triglycerides (fasting blood test/every 5 years or more often as needed)

❑ Serum creatinine/eGFR (blood test/once a year)

❑ Urine albumin-to-creatinine ratio (urine sample/once a year)

What to Bring with You

When you make your appointment, ask your diabetes care provider, nurse, or the office receptionist what to bring with you. Every office and provider is a little bit different, so it never hurts to ask.

Typically, you'll bring along your blood glucose meter or logbook so you and your provider can discuss how your numbers look. Your provider may like to see these numbers as a printout, or she may have the software to download the numbers from your meter to a spreadsheet in her office.

You may find it easiest to put all your medications into a plastic bag and bring them with you to your office visit. That way, you won't forget any medications or their doses. You can also use your smartphone to take a photo of all your medications to show your physician. Ideally, your physician should have all your medications recorded in your chart, but she may not if other specialists write prescriptions for you. Bring the physical bottles or take a photo so everything can be recorded and up to date during your exam.

Don't forget to bring a list of your questions or concerns to your checkup. It can be easy to forget issues if you only see your provider twice a year. Keep a notebook in your kitchen, bedroom, or living room so you can write down questions as they pop into your head. Bring a pen so you can jot down answers or tips for finding out more information online or in books.

Here's a handy checklist of items to take to your doctor appointment so you don't forget anything:

- ❑ Blood glucose meter or logbook
- ❑ A list of your medications
- ❑ List of questions and concerns and a pen to take notes

Communicating like a Pro

Communication is so important when working with your healthcare team. Check that all your providers have one another's names, phone numbers, and fax numbers so they can share your health records or call each other if something comes up. Make sure all the providers on your team know when you make changes to your medications or other treatments. It's also helpful for everyone to know if you make lifestyle changes like quitting smoking or beginning a new weight-loss diet.

Your team is there to support you, so don't be shy to lean on them when you have questions or concerns. You may need to take the initiative to contact a team member, especially if you don't have a regularly scheduled exam anytime soon. The next time you have an appointment, ask your provider how he or she likes to handle questions. Should you email, call, talk to a nurse on staff, or just make an appointment? Every office is different, so ask ahead of time about the best way to communicate when you have questions.

It may seem intimidating to put yourself out there and raise a concern. After all, everybody feels nervous and worried asking about things they don't know or think they should know. *Remember:* Part of your role as the leader of your healthcare team is to voice your concerns and feelings so your providers can offer helpful solutions and treatments.

TIP

Use the following tips to help you feel more comfortable talking to your diabetes care provider or CDE about your questions and concerns:

>> Write down your questions ahead of time and bring that paper with you. Be prepared by bringing along your meter and/or logbook and a list of your current medications.

>> Start your appointment by telling your provider what you hope to accomplish and asking her what she hopes to accomplish during this visit.

>> If you don't understand something, ask again. Diabetes is a chronic condition with lots of moving parts like diet, exercise, medications, and monitoring. It's normal not to understand everything all at once and totally okay to ask for clarification.

>> Bring a notebook and write your doctor's instructions down as you go, if that's helpful. It won't offend your provider, and might even encourage her that you're listening and ready to take action when you get home.

One of the most important steps you'll take with your diabetes care provider, or really any provider, is to set goals. Make sure you clearly understand your goals and talk about the specific action steps you'll take to achieve those goals. For example, if you want to lose 5 pounds, talk about each step you'll take along the way, such as eating smaller portions or exercising an extra day a week.

Another part of achieving goals is measuring your progress. Talk about how you'll measure your progress in your daily life. After all, you're the one living with diabetes 365 days a year, not just during the hour spent in your provider's office. Talk about how you'll measure successes and tweak your challenges to achieve each one of your goals. Measuring goals could include keeping a logbook of blood glucose readings, writing down meal specifics, or starting a journal to record your feelings and mood.

Chapter **5**

Diabetes Education Classes

A diabetes education class may be your first opportunity to really learn what diabetes is and how it will affect your body. When you find out you have type 2 diabetes, the only thing you may be able to focus on is the diagnosis. You may feel disbelief, shock, or dread. You may feel numb at the prospect of living with a chronic disease. Instead of asking a lot of questions, you may feel overwhelmed, which may discourage you from finding out much about diabetes. This is totally natural.

Don't beat yourself up. You have plenty of opportunity to educate yourself and ask all your questions during diabetes education classes and training. A diabetes education class is a chance for you to learn all about diabetes and how to care for yourself. In addition to taking classes, you'll have the option to brush up on your knowledge or learn new behaviors during annual or as-needed consultations. Read on to find out more about diabetes education, what you can expect, and how to find a class in your area.

Getting Informed about Diabetes Education

Diabetes education is simply an opportunity to increase your knowledge of diabetes and skills for managing diabetes during your everyday life. Diabetes education is often referred to as *diabetes self-management education and support* (DSME/S).

The most well-known type of diabetes education is probably a *diabetes education class*, which is often taught in a group setting by a diabetes educator (see Chapter 3 for more about diabetes educators). However, diabetes education can also refer to annual visits with your healthcare team to assess your needs. You may also be referred for diabetes education if you have complications or changes that affect how you take care of yourself.

As part of diabetes education, you'll learn about healthy eating strategies. Most people on your healthcare team should be able to answer questions that arise. However, there may be times when you're referred to a registered dietitian nutritionist or other specialist to learn more. (Flip to Chapter 11 to find out more about dietitians and how to be reimbursed for these visits.)

In addition, you'll learn coping skills for managing the common emotional concerns that can go along with having a chronic condition. Yet, you may ask for a referral to a mental health professional if you feel like you need additional support. See more about finding support in Chapter 15.

When do I go?

There are four critical times to take part in diabetes education:

» When you're first diagnosed with diabetes

» During an annual visit with your healthcare team

» If you experience complications (such as change in vision) that affect how you take care of your diabetes

» If you experience transitions (such as a change in your living situation) that affect how you take care of yourself

Diagnosis is perhaps the most critical time to attend a diabetes education class. You'll learn the basics of taking care of your blood glucose and preventing complications. Find out more about the topics these classes address in the upcoming section "Knowing What to Expect."

Your annual visit with your healthcare team is another opportunity to enhance your diabetes education. Your diabetes care provider will ask you specific questions about how you're managing your diabetes and whether you need help in specific areas. For example, you may be asked about your insulin regimen or whether you're incorporating healthy foods into your meals. Your provider may refer you to a diabetes educator, dietitian, or other specialist to focus on learning new skills or changing behaviors.

Diabetes education can improve your health. Some studies have shown that diabetes self-management and education can improve A1C by as much as 1 percent.

Complications can arise at any time, so consider these within the context of your everyday care. For example, you may have changes in your health such as kidney disease, a stroke, or a complicated new medication regimen that could impact your diabetes care. You may also encounter changes in your vision, your dexterity, or even your movement that might impact your diabetes care. Don't discount mental and emotional changes such as anxiety or depression, which can impact your motivation and ability to take care of yourself.

If you experience any of these or other complications, talk to your diabetes care provider about how they will impact your daily self-care routine. If you have concerns, ask for a referral to a diabetes educator or other specialist to help manage complications.

Likewise, transitions can occur at any time, and sometimes out of nowhere. For example, your living situation may change and you may now live alone or be moving to an assisted-living facility. Transitions could also occur when your healthcare team changes or when changes in health insurance necessitate a significant medication change. Sometimes, just getting older is enough of a transition to spark a refresh of your diabetes education.

Meeting the educator

The most obvious providers of diabetes education are diabetes educators. Diabetes educators are specially trained to help you manage your diabetes. They can help you learn how to take new medications, incorporate new foods into your meals, or start getting more physically active no matter how sedentary you've been in the past.

When you enroll in a diabetes education class (tips for finding a class are discussed later in this chapter), look for diabetes educators who have one of the following certifications:

>> **Certified diabetes educator (CDE):** This certification is given to a healthcare professional who has sufficiently completed the required number of hours in clinical practice, passed an exam from the National Certification Board for Diabetes Educators, and directly oversees patients in diabetes education. It could be a nurse, pharmacist, dietitian, physician, physician assistant (PA), or other provider.

>> **Board certified-advanced diabetes management (BC-ADM):** The American Association of Diabetes Educators (AADE) offers this certification for advanced level practitioners. A BC-ADM can adjust medications, treat complications, and address psychosocial issues, among other skills.

If you can't find someone with these credentials, it's not the end of the world. Diabetes education can come from any knowledgeable member of your healthcare team. You can always learn something new about diabetes!

Knowing What to Expect

Diabetes education is a cornerstone of your diabetes management. Why is it so darned important? Because you're the one who's taking care of your diabetes most of the time. It's not your doctor or nurse or dietitian or spouse. The most important person is you. And you can only be effective if you understand what diabetes is and how it affects your body.

At the heart of diabetes education are both coping skills and behaviors that will help you navigate a chronic condition. You don't get a day off when you have diabetes, so you'll need all the tools in the box (and beyond) to get you through the days, weeks, and years ahead.

It's not a one-size-fits-all education because caring for your diabetes is not a one-size-fits-all prescription. Instead, diabetes education should address your current knowledge, cultural preferences, emotional concerns, financial constraints, medical history, and physical limitations.

Diabetes education at diagnosis

When you're first diagnosed with type 2 diabetes, your provider will likely refer you to a diabetes education class. Usually the class takes place over 2 sessions or more, sometimes spread out over several weeks. The class could take place in a hospital or private practice or other location (see the "Finding a class in your area" section later in this chapter for more details).

During this class you'll find out what diabetes is and how it affects your body. You'll probably discuss all the things we touch on in Chapter 1, like your pancreas, beta cells, and insulin.

You'll probably learn how to check your blood glucose using a meter and test strips. It may be the first time you've ever pricked your own finger for a blood sample. Don't be nervous. The diabetes educator is on hand to guide you through the step-by-step process. (Find out more about checking your blood glucose in Chapter 7.)

This initial class is also an ideal time to find out about common complications of diabetes, such as blood vessel and nerve damage, and how to prevent and treat them (see Chapter 8). Your diabetes educator may talk about different types of medications, including how they work and potential side effects (see Chapter 6).

Perhaps most important, you'll learn essential actions for making healthy choices such as eating wholesome, nutritious foods and controlling portions, adding more physical activity to your daily life, and stopping unhealthy behaviors like smoking.

In addition to a class, you may have a follow-up visit with a diabetes educator to discuss individual concerns or develop personalized goals or plans moving forward.

Traditionally, these classes are open to spouses or other loved ones, who are part of your support system. If you think that might be helpful, call ahead and ask if you can bring a family member or friend to your class. Another set of eyes and ears can be beneficial when you're learning about diabetes care.

Also, you may just meet someone like you at a diabetes education class. After all, you're in a class with others with type 2 diabetes learning about the same topics and sharing similar concerns and questions. This can be a positive experience. Developing an informal network of friends from a diabetes education class is a perk.

TIP

Digital diabetes education is on the horizon, and recently the American Diabetes Association recognized the first digital program. Called One Drop-Experts, it's a mobile app that offers scalable diabetes education and coaching.

Keeping up with diabetes developments

A diabetes class is not a one-and-done experience. Diabetes education is part of your ongoing management and support. You may go to initial classes after your diagnosis of type 2 diabetes, and then visit a diabetes educator every year to revisit your diabetes management goals and prevent complications. Seek out support for managing your diabetes if you have new complicating factors like depression, changes in dexterity, or totally new medications. Diabetes education and support can help you navigate these changes so that you can cope more effectively and prevent complications.

Finding a class in your area

It used to be that diabetes education typically took place in a formal setting, like a hospital, soon after patients were diagnosed by their provider. This is the typical diabetes education class that many people with type 2 diabetes still experience today.

Yet, you may find that your diabetes education takes a different form. For example, your diabetes care provider's office may offer its own diabetes education classes. Or you may take a diabetes education class at a medical or assisted-living home where you live. Community health centers and pharmacies also offer diabetes education. You may take part in diabetes education as part of a shared-office visit in which you and several patients have a group appointment. Lastly, you can get diabetes education online or through a video conference.

REMEMBER

Diabetes self-management education saves money, too! Studies show that this education reduces hospital admissions and readmissions and healthcare costs because of lower risks of complications from diabetes. And diabetes education classes are usually covered by insurance.

If your diabetes care provider gave you information about a class or the name of a diabetes educator, then you're one step ahead. You just need to make the call to get started!

However, if you're uncertain whom to call, then ask your provider or other member of your healthcare team for a referral or recommendation. You can also call your local hospital or community health clinic to find classes in your area.

TIP

Both the American Diabetes Association and the American Association of Diabetes Educators have resources and online tools for locating diabetes education programs in your neighborhood. Visit www.diabeteseducator.org for a listing of accredited diabetes education programs run by either organization.

Receiving diabetes education through telehealth may be a good option for people who live in rural parts of the United States, have mobility issues, or don't have access to classes or educators in their area. Medicare offers tele-education in some areas. Telehealth allows you to connect with a diabetes educator via real-time audio and video.

Investigating Insurance Coverage for the Cost of Classes

Individual health insurance often pays for diabetes education. For example, "insurance plans typically cover up to 10 hours of diabetes education the first year you have been referred, with varying levels of coverage after that," according to the AADE website.

Call the number on your health insurance card to find out more about your benefits, including details about amounts or number of hours covered. You may need a referral from your provider, and these services may need to be provided by someone who is certified and registered for this training, so ask about this, too.

Medicare Part B covers diabetes education (called *diabetes self-management training*, or DSMT). "It includes tips for eating healthy, being active, monitoring blood sugar, taking drugs, and reducing risks," according to the Medicare.gov website. It may cover up to 10 hours of initial diabetes education, including 1 hour of individual training and 9 hours of group training. And you could also qualify for 2 hours of follow-up training each year, according to the website. You'll need a written order from your healthcare provider.

Despite all the benefits of diabetes education, studies show that not enough people take advantage of these classes and training. A 2014 report from the Centers for Disease Control and Prevention found that less than 7 percent of people with diabetes with private insurance participated in diabetes education in the first year after diagnosis.

Chapter **6**

Medications and Surgery

Your lifestyle choices are incredibly important when you have type 2 diabetes. Eating wholesome, nutritious foods and staying physically active are cornerstones of managing your blood glucose. Some people, particularly soon after diagnosis, can manage their diabetes solely by making changes to their lifestyle like eating healthy foods and exercising regularly. They probably lose a few pounds, too. It's inspiring that these healthy choices can be so impactful! (You can find out more about eating healthy foods and moving more in Part 4.)

Most people with type 2 diabetes need to take medications, in addition to making lifestyle changes, to manage their blood glucose. If you need to take a diabetes medication, you are certainly not alone.

No single medication is used to treat everyone with type 2 diabetes. Instead, quite a few classes of medications are used to treat diabetes, and each class features different brands. Medications include pills you take by mouth, medications you inject once a day or once a week, and of course, insulin.

New medications for type 2 diabetes are constantly being developed; many more medications are available today than, say, 20 years ago. Some old medications work incredibly well, and others have fallen out of favor because of side effects.

This chapter describes each type of medication — how it works, how you take it, and possible side effects and precautions.

Besides medications specifically targeted at blood glucose, you might take medications for your blood pressure and cholesterol. You also find out about these commonly used pills in this chapter. And don't forget surgery: It's now a recommended treatment option for some people with type 2 diabetes.

Why Do I Need to Take Medication?

People with type 2 diabetes have several things going on in their bodies with blood glucose, insulin, and other hormones:

>> People with type 2 diabetes may not make as much insulin as they used to — or none at all.

>> People with type 2 diabetes may not be as sensitive to the hormone insulin (called *insulin resistance*) as people who don't have diabetes.

>> Other hormones, called incretins, affect how much insulin the body releases and help control blood glucose. For some people with type 2 diabetes, a hormone called *glucagon-like peptide-1* (GLP-1) may not work properly and may not stimulate the pancreas to make enough insulin.

>> People with type 2 diabetes may release too much glucose from their livers, causing blood glucose to rise.

All these things can cause high blood glucose, which can cause short- and long-term health problems. (Read more about the complications of type 2 diabetes in Chapter 8.) Medication can target these different problems to help lower your blood glucose. In this chapter, we describe how each medication works. Some people with type 2 diabetes may need to take insulin because their bodies are no longer responsive to blood glucose–lowering medications or because their bodies don't make any insulin at all.

REMEMBER

Your diabetes medication regimen can change over time. You may take a drug like metformin at the beginning, but then need to add or change medications to keep your blood glucose in your target range later on. (*Remember:* Most people are aiming for an A1C of 7 percent or less.) Or you may experience side effects that prompt medication changes. You may also need to take insulin at diagnosis or several years down the road. It totally depends on the individual!

Your healthcare team is your number-one resource for medications. You'll work with your nurse, doctor, pharmacist, physician assistant, or diabetes educator to troubleshoot problems or adjust doses.

WARNING

Never stop taking a medication because you think it's not working or because of annoying *side effects* (an unintended effect, such as diarrhea or flatulence, of taking a certain drug). Instead, call your provider and tell her what's going on. Don't be shy about bringing up concerns like bowel movements, changes in mood, or any other concern. All drugs can have side effects, although some may be more severe than others.

TIP

Know the names, doses, and instructions for each medication you take. If you're like most people, you'll probably need to write them down. Don't be afraid to ask your provider or pharmacist for these details each time you see her.

Pills for Type 2 Diabetes

The majority of medications for type 2 diabetes are oral medications, meaning they're in pill form. Some have been around for decades, and others have recently been approved by the Food and Drug Administration (FDA). Pills for type 2 diabetes fall into nine major *classes*, which is just a fancy way of saying that these groups of medications work in similar ways. Within each class, there are usually generic and brand-name versions of medications in the class. You'll also find combination pills that combine two different medications into one dose.

TIP

Ask your provider about potential side effects whenever you start taking a new medication. Then keep an eye out for these problems and call your doctor if you notice anything out of the ordinary.

REMEMBER

Tell your provider if you're thinking about becoming pregnant, because some type 2 diabetes medications are not recommended during pregnancy.

Supplements, including vitamins or herbal remedies, and certain foods can interfere with your medications. Over-the-counter medications can also impact prescription drugs. Tell your provider about any supplements or over-the-counter medications you're currently taking and how you normally take them with meals.

Table 6-1 lists the oral medications for type 2 diabetes. The following sections cover these medications in greater detail.

TABLE 6-1 **Oral Medications for Type 2 Diabetes**

Drug Class	How It Works	Generic Name	Brand Name
Biguanides	Improves sensitivity to glucose. Blocks the release of glucose from the liver.	Metformin	Glucophage
Sulfonylureas	Stimulates your body to produce more insulin. Helps to lower your blood glucose after meals.	Glimepiride	Amaryl (and various generics)
		Glipizide	Glucotrol, Glucotrol XL (and various generics)
		Glyburide	Micronase, DiaBeta, Glynase PresTab (and various generics)
Meglitinides	Stimulates your body to produce more insulin.	Repaglinide	Prandin
		Nateglinide	Starlix
Dipeptidyl-peptidase 4 (DPP-4) inhibitors	Keeps the blood glucose–lowering hormone glucagon-like peptide-1 (GLP-1) in your body.	Sitagliptin	Januvia
		Saxagliptin	Onglyza
		Linagliptin	Tradjenta
		Alogliptin	Nesina
Sodium-glucose cotransporter 2 (SGLT2) inhibitors	Blocks glucose from being reabsorbed by the kidneys. Helps your body excrete excess glucose through your urine.	Canagliflozin	Invokana
		Dapagliflozin	Farxiga
		Empagliflozin	Jardiance
Alpha-glucosidase inhibitors	Slows the digestion of the carbohydrates you eat.	Acarbose	Precose (and various generics)
		Miglitol	Glyset (and various generics)
Thiazolidinediones (TZDs)	Improves sensitivity to glucose.	Pioglitazone	Actos
		Rosiglitazone	Avandia
Bile acid sequestrants	Binds to bile acids in the intestines to lower blood glucose and cholesterol.	Colesevelam	Welchol
Dopamine-2 agonist	Lowers blood glucose in some people with type 2 diabetes.	Bromocriptine	Cycloset

Biguanides

Biguanides improve the body's sensitivity to insulin and block the release of glucose from the liver. Biguanides include the most commonly prescribed medication for type 2 diabetes: metformin. Yes, you've probably heard this name before. There's a reason it's popular: It's safe, effective, and inexpensive for many people.

Metformin is often the first medication prescribed to patients diagnosed with type 2 diabetes. And it can even be prescribed to prevent diabetes in people at risk for the disease (with a diagnosis of *prediabetes*).

Metformin was approved in the United States in the 1990s under the brand name Glucophage. Now, the generic form, called metformin, is readily available. You take metformin as a pill, usually two times a day. It's also available as a liquid. Glucophage XR is an extended-release version that is also available generically.

Metformin doesn't improve your body's ability to make insulin, so it's unlikely to cause episodes of low blood glucose, which is a good thing. It does have some side effects; the most common is diarrhea or loose stools. Other side effects like nausea can occur, too. Tell your healthcare provider about any side effects so she can work with you to adjust the dose or change medications.

WARNING

A rare but serious side effect of metformin in certain patients is called *lactic acidosis*, which can cause muscle pain and weakness and other symptoms. People with severe kidney disease should not take metformin.

TIP

Ask your provider about vitamin B12 deficiency if you've been taking metformin for a long time. He may measure your B12 levels and, if they're low, recommend taking a vitamin B12 supplement.

Sulfonylureas

Sulfonylureas help you make more insulin and lower your blood glucose after meals. Sulfonylureas include glimepiride (Amaryl and various generics), glipizide (Glucotrol, Gluctorol XL, and various generics), and glyburide (Micronase, DiaBeta, Glynase PresTab, and various generics).

Sulfonylureas were first approved in the 1950s, and they're often taken once or twice a day.

Each type of sulfonylurea has different dosing, side effects, and interactions with other drugs. Sulfonylureas stimulate your body to produce insulin, so they can cause low blood glucose. Some of the most common side effects across all sulfonylureas are episodes of low blood glucose, weight gain, and skin rashes.

Meglitinides

Meglitinides help you make more insulin and lower your blood glucose. They include repaglinide (Prandin) and nateglinade (Starlix). They're similar to sulfonylureas but faster acting.

Repaglinide was approved in 1997 and Nateglinide was approved in 2000. Meglitinides work quickly and for about 4 hours. They're taken three times a day, just before meals.

Meglitinides can cause episodes of low blood glucose, weight gain, nausea or vomiting, and headaches.

Dipeptidyl-peptidase 4 (DPP-4) inhibitors

DPP-4 inhibitors work by keeping the "helpful hormone" GLP-1 around in your body. GLP-1 naturally lowers blood glucose, but your body breaks down GLP-1 quickly. DPP-4 inhibitors stop that breakdown and lower blood glucose. DPP-4 inhibitors include sitagliptin (Januvia), saxagliptin (Onglyza), linagliptin (Tradjenta), and alogliptin (Nesina).

Sitagliptin was the first DPP-4 inhibitor approved in the United States in 2006. DPP-4 inhibitors are usually taken once a day.

DPP-4 inhibitors can cause side effects like upper respiratory infections, sore throats, and headaches. They may also cause joint pain that is severe and disabling. And they may cause inflammation of the pancreas, which can cause gastrointestinal symptoms like pain in the abdomen, nausea, or vomiting. Tell your healthcare provider if you've noticed any of these side effects.

TECHNICAL STUFF

Incretins are a group of hormones that signal the body to release insulin after eating. Scientists have developed medications that target these hormones for people with type 2 diabetes. Two medications, DPP-4 inhibitors (pill) and GLP-1 agonists (injectable), work by regulating these hormones.

Sodium-glucose cotransporter 2 (SGLT2) inhibitors

Sodium-glucose cotransporter 2 (SGLT2) inhibitors work differently from the medications covered earlier. They block your kidneys from reabsorbing glucose into your bloodstream and help you excrete excess glucose through your urine. In this way, SGLT2 inhibitors lower blood glucose. They can also help you lose weight. Also, SGLT2 inhibitors could benefit patients at a high risk for cardiovascular disease. These medications include canagliflozin (Invokana), dapagliflozin (Farxiga), and empagliflozin (Jardiance).

Canagliflozin was approved in 2013; dapagliflozin and empagliflozin were approved in 2014. They're taken once a day.

SGLT2 inhibitors can cause urinary tract and genital yeast infections and increased urination leading to dehydration. Canagliflozin and dapagliflozin carry a risk for kidney injury. In rare cases, canagliflozin causes an increased risk of leg and foot amputations, according to two large clinical trials.

Alpha-glucosidase inhibitors

Alpha-glucosidase inhibitors also work a little differently from other medications. They slow down your digestion of carbohydrates during meals and lower blood glucose. They include acarbose (Precose and various generics) and miglitol (Glyset and various generics).

Alpha-glucosidase inhibitors were approved in the mid-1990s. They're taken three times a day at the beginning of each meal.

Side effects include gas, stomach pain, and diarrhea. They can also contribute to episodes of low blood glucose, and because these medications can slow the breakdown of sugars such as fruit juice, always use a glucose product such as glucose gel to treat symptoms of hypoglycemia.

Thiazolidinediones (TZDs)

Thiazolidinediones (TZDs) make you more sensitive to insulin and lower blood glucose. They include pioglitazone (Actos) and rosiglitazone (Avandia).

TZDs were approved in the late 1990s. They're taken once or twice a day.

Side effects of TZDs have made them less commonly prescribed, particularly rosiglitazone. In 2010, the FDA imposed restrictions for prescribing rosiglitazone because of concern over increased cardiovascular risk, although those restrictions were lifted in 2013. Rosiglitazone may also increase the risk of bone fractures. Pioglitazone may increase the risk of bladder cancer; people with a history of bladder cancer should not use it. Other side effects include headache, sore throat, and back pain.

Bile acid sequestrants

Bile acid sequestrants bind to bile acids in the intestinal tract and lower blood glucose and cholesterol. There is one with FDA approval called colesevelam (Welchol).

Side effects include gas, constipation, nausea, diarrhea, stomach pain, and weakness or muscle pain.

Dopamine-2 agonists

Dopamine-2 agonists lower blood glucose in some people with type 2 diabetes, although how they work is unclear. One medication, bromocriptine (Cycloset), is FDA approved for this use.

Side effects include dizziness, nausea, and fatigue.

Combination pills for type 2 diabetes

Your provider may recommend a combination pill if your body needs more help lowering blood glucose. A combination pill is handy because you only need to take one, versus two or more pills, at a time. Some common examples of combination pills include

>> Metformin and glipizide (Metaglip)

>> Metformin and glyburide (Glucovance)

>> Metformin and sitagliptin (Janumet and Janumet XR)

>> Metformin and linagliptin (Jentadueto and Jentadueto XR)

>> Metformin and repaglinide (Prandimet)

>> Metformin, extended release, and saxagliptin (Kombiglyze XR)

>> Metformin and alogliptin (Kazano)

>> Metformin, extended release, and dapagliflozin (Xigduo XR)

>> Metformin and canagliflozin (Invokamet and Invokamet XR)

>> Metformin and empagliflozin (Synjardy and Synjardy XR)

>> Metformin and pioglitazone (ActosPlus Met and ActosPlus Met XR)

>> Metformin and rosiglitazone (Avandamet)

>> Dapagliflozin and saxagliptin (Qtern)

>> Empagliflozin and linagliptin (Glyxambi)

>> Glimepiride and pioglitazone (Duetact)

>> Glimepiride and rosiglitazone (Avandaryl)

>> Alogliptin and pioglitazone (Oseni)

Injected Medications for Type 2 Diabetes (Besides Insulin)

Pills aren't the only option for people to lower their blood glucose (see the preceding section). Now patients have access to injected medications (other than insulin), which are injected under the skin with a needle. This is different from a pill that you pop in your mouth.

There are two non-insulin classes of injected medication for type 2 diabetes: GLP-1 agonists and amylin analogs.

Table 6-2 lists the injected medications for type 2 diabetes. The following sections cover these medications in greater detail.

TABLE 6-2   **Injected Medications for Type 2 Diabetes**

Drug Class	How It Works	Generic Name	Brand Name
Glucagon-like peptide-1 (GLP-1) receptor agonists	Mimics the action of the incretin hormone GLP-1. Stimulates your body to produce more insulin. Slows down how quickly your stomach empties.	Exenatide	Byetta
		Extended Release Exenatide	Bydureon
		Liraglutide	Victoza
		Dulaglutide	Trulicity
		Lixisenatide	Adlyxin
Amylin analogs	Mimics the action of the hormone amylin. Slows down how quickly your stomach empties. Suppresses your liver from releasing glucagon, a hormone that moves glucose into your bloodstream.	Pramlintide	Symlin

GLP-1 agonists

Glucagon-like peptide-1 receptor agonists (wow, that's a mouthful) are otherwise know as GLP-1 agonists. They're also sometimes called incretin mimetics because they mimic the action of the incretin hormone GLP-1, which helps lower blood glucose. GLP-1 agonists help your body make more insulin and slow down how quickly your stomach empties so your blood glucose doesn't rise as rapidly. They may also make you less hungry and encourage some weight loss. GLP-1 agonists include exenatide (Byetta), liraglutide (Victoza), extended-release exenatide (Bydureon), dulaglutide (Trulicity), and lixisenatide (Adlyxin). Victoza can be used to reduce the risk of heart attack, stroke, and other cardiovascular events in adults with type 2 diabetes and at high risk for cardiovascular disease.

Exenatide received FDA approval in 2005. You inject GLP-1 agonists using a pre-dosed pen. Depending on the medication, you may inject twice a day, once a day, or once a week.

Side effects include weight loss, nausea and vomiting (and resulting dehydration), episodes of low blood glucose, kidney problems, and inflammation of the pancreas. Tell your healthcare provider if you've had pancreatitis, gallstones, a history of alcoholism, high triglycerides, or kidney problems.

TIP

Whether you're starting a new medication or just can't remember, don't be afraid to ask your healthcare provider why you're taking it. Knowing the reasons *why* you take a specific medication may help you remember to take it — or just feel more empowered about your actions.

Amylin analogs

Amylin analogs mimic a hormone called amylin that the body naturally produces along with insulin. Pramlintide (Symlin) is a manufactured version of this hormone. Some people with type 2 diabetes don't make enough insulin or enough amylin. Pramlintide lowers blood glucose by slowing how fast your stomach empties and suppressing your liver from releasing a hormone called glucagon, which puts glucose into your bloodstream. It may also encourage you to eat less because you feel more full at meals.

Pramlintide received FDA approval in 2005 for people with type 1 or type 2 diabetes who use insulin. You inject pramlintide using a disposable pen during meals. It does not replace insulin. It's helpful for people who need something beyond insulin to help control their blood glucose.

Side effects include episodes of low blood glucose, nausea, vomiting, stomach pain, and headache.

All About Insulin

Insulin is that all-important hormone that helps us get energy from the foods we eat. Insulin does that by letting glucose into cells. Without insulin, glucose stays in the bloodstream and leads to high blood glucose. High blood glucose can make you feel crummy in the short term, but it can also lead to long-term complications like heart disease, stroke, and kidney disease.

Insulin is also a medication for type 2 diabetes. We've put the topic of insulin into its own section in this chapter because there is a lot of information to cover. You find out the basics of insulin therapy, types of insulin, and how it's delivered and stored.

There is not one single *reason* why people with type 2 diabetes take insulin. Some people need to take insulin because changes to their foods, physical activity, or medications cannot lower their blood glucose. Some people need to take insulin because they're allergic to other medications. Some people may take insulin when they become pregnant.

There also is not one single *time* when people with type 2 diabetes take insulin. Some people take insulin when they're first diagnosed with type 2 diabetes. Some people take insulin after they've had diabetes for years or decades. Some people with type 2 diabetes may never need to take insulin.

TIP

Never look at starting insulin as a failure. It is not a judgment. It is not good or bad. Instead, taking insulin is just doing what you need to take care of your body.

Insulin 101

Insulin is a naturally occurring hormone in your body. However, insulin also refers to the man-made, manufactured medication that people with diabetes use in order to survive and live healthy lives.

For a person without diabetes, the body produces insulin naturally. It releases a low, background level throughout the day and night, as well as bursts of insulin during meals to manage those carbs! A person without diabetes doesn't feel or experience a thing related to insulin. It just happens as part of the body's everyday workings. The body naturally releases insulin to keep blood glucose within a range of about 60–100 mg/dL while fasting and 140 mg/dL or less after eating.

Insulin therapy

People with diabetes who take insulin are trying to mimic the body's natural way of releasing insulin. However, it's not as straightforward as you might expect. It takes special formulations, delivery, and timing of insulin to get close.

Insulin therapy is a fancy name for giving yourself insulin. Insulin therapy may require one or several different forms of insulin to simulate the background release and bursts of insulin that naturally occur in the body of people without diabetes. Insulin comes in different types, mixtures, and strengths. You inject this insulin at different times too. The way you inject insulin can also vary; you may need to use a needle, pen, pump, or inhaler.

Basal (background) and bolus insulin therapy

Basal insulin mimics the background level of insulin in the body. It's the steady, low stream that occurs between eating during the day and while you're sleeping at night. Basal insulin is an intermediate- or long-acting insulin that is absorbed slowly.

Bolus insulin mimics the bursts of insulin that occur in your body. You'll need bolus insulin when you eat something and you need to process those carbohydrates for energy. This is called a mealtime bolus. It is an extra amount of insulin taken to cover an expected rise in blood glucose.

Some people with type 2 diabetes need just basal insulin, or that steady, low background level. For example, you may take basal insulin in the morning or at night or both. Some people with type 2 diabetes need just bolus insulin, or those short bursts. Still others need both basal and bolus insulin therapy.

Types of insulin

People with diabetes have been able to inject insulin since the 1920s when scientists began extracting insulin from the pancreases of cows and pigs. Phew, we've come a long way in the last century! Since the 1980s, pharmaceutical companies have been able to manufacture synthetic human insulin.

Nowadays, two groups of injected insulin are available: synthetic human insulin and analog insulin. Within these two groups of insulin, there are different types that have varying characteristics regarding when they start to work, when they peak, and how long they last.

Hopefully, your eyes haven't started to glaze over yet, because there is plenty more information to cover about insulin. It may seem like a lot to digest at first, but you'll soon get the hang of it. *Remember:* Your healthcare team is your best source for questions about insulin. No one is going to just give you a needle and a bottle of insulin and say, "Good luck."

Instead, you'll come up with an insulin plan — with the help of your healthcare provider, of course — for your type(s) of insulin, including when, how much, and how often to use insulin. This section is meant to be a primer so you know the scope of options available.

Table 6-3 lists the commonly used types of insulin. The following sections cover these medications in greater detail.

Human insulin

Synthetic human insulin is manufactured to be the same chemical structure as the insulin that your body naturally produces. However, its action is not the same as your body's insulin because it clumps up when you inject it under the skin and it takes longer to absorb.

There are three types of human insulin:

» **Short-acting human insulin** (also called regular insulin) starts to work in 30 minutes, peaks at 2–3 hours, and lasts for 5–8 hours.

» **Intermediate-acting insulin** (also called NPH) starts to work in 2–4 hours, peaks at 4–10 hours, and lasts for 10–16 hours.

» **Premixed combinations** of short- and intermediate-acting insulin are also available.

TECHNICAL STUFF

How is human insulin made? Scientists put the human gene for insulin into bacteria or yeast, causing them to churn out insulin. The insulin is then extracted and purified. *Voilá!* It's human insulin, without the humans (or perhaps a little help from humans).

Analog insulin

Analog insulin is manufactured to be similar to human insulin, but it has certain more desirable traits such as working more quickly or more slowly. Analog insulin is newer than human insulin — and it's also more expensive.

TABLE 6-3 **Commonly Used Insulin Types and Action Profiles**

Type of Insulin	Generic Name	Brand Name	Onset	Peak	Duration
Fast-acting insulin	Insulin glulisine	Apidra	15 minutes	1–2 hours	3–5 hours
	Insulin lispro	Humalog			
	Insulin aspart	Novolog			
	Inhaled insulin	Afrezza			
Regular/short-acting insulin	Regular insulin	Humulin R	30 minutes	2–3 hours	5–8 hours
		Novolin R			
Intermediate-acting insulin	NPH insulin	Humulin N	2–4 hours	4–10 hours	10–16 hours
		Novolin N			
Long-acting insulin	Insulin detemir	Levemir	1–2 hours	No peak	Up to 24+ hours (up to 42 hours for insulin degludec)
	Insulin glargine	Lantus			
		Basaglar			
	Insulin degludec	Tresiba			
Premixed insulin	70% NPH/30% regular	Humulin 70/30	30 minutes	2–12 hours	18–24 hours
		Novolin 70/30	30 minutes	2–12 hours	18–24 hours
	50% lispro protamine (NPL)/50% lispro	Humalog Mix 50/50	15–30 minutes	1–5 hours	14–24 hours
	75% lispro protamine (NPL)/25% lispro	Humalog Mix 75/25	15–30 minutes	1–6.5 hours	14–24 hours
	70% aspart protamine/30% aspart	Novolog Mix 70/30	10–20 minutes	1–4 hours	18–24 hours

There are three types of analog insulin:

» **Fast-acting insulin** starts to work in 15 minutes, peaks in 1–2 hours, and lasts for 3–5 hours.

» **Long-acting insulin** starts to work in 1–2 hours and can last up to 24 hours.

» **Premixed analog insulin** starts to work in 5–15 minutes and lasts up to 24 hours.

Whether you take human or analog insulin depends on many factors such as cost (in general, human insulin is cheaper), insurance coverage, convenience (analogs can provide more flexibility), and your blood glucose goals.

Inhaled insulin

Afrezza is the only FDA-approved inhaled insulin. Adults without chronic lung problems may be eligible to use Afrezza. You use an inhaler to breathe in Afrezza during mealtimes. It's a fast-acting insulin that starts working within 15 minutes, peaks at about 1 hour, and last for 3 hours.

Buying and storing insulin

Your healthcare provider will give you a prescription for insulin, which will usually come in a vial. Read the package instructions about the best way to store insulin once you get it from the pharmacy. Usually, insulin can be kept at room temperature for up to a month. And that's the preferred way to do it because injecting insulin at room temperature is more comfortable than injecting cold insulin. Unopened vials of insulin can be stored in the refrigerator.

Never expose insulin to extreme temperatures like the freezer or the hot sun (or inside your car on a summer day). These changes in temperature could affect its potency. Also check the expiration date just like you would with any other medication. Don't use insulin if it's expired. Instead, return it to your pharmacy.

Also, inspect the insulin before you inject it. Visual cues are helpful. Rapid-acting, long-acting, and regular insulin should be clear without floating pieces. Intermediate-acting and premixed insulin should be cloudy, but also without floating pieces or crystals. If you suspect anything funky, don't use the insulin, and take it back to your pharmacist for concerns or a refund or exchange.

Insulin prices have been steadily increasing, making it difficult for some people without health insurance (or with limited health insurance) to afford medications. Insulin manufacturers have special programs to help lower-income individuals obtain insulin. Insulin affordability is a major advocacy issue for the American Diabetes Association.

Injecting insulin: Syringes, pens, and more

You can inject insulin using a syringe or an insulin pen. We cover insulin infusion in the following section on insulin pumps. Whether you choose a syringe or pen for your insulin is a matter of personal preference.

All about insulin syringes

Many people use syringes to inject insulin. They've been around for ages! Syringes are made of a disposable plastic tube with a needle on the end. You insert the needle into a vial of insulin and draw up the insulin into the syringe (see Figure 6-1). Syringes hold a variety of insulin amounts or doses, so choose a syringe that holds your entire dose of insulin. For example, if you take a 40-unit dose, don't choose a 30-unit syringe.

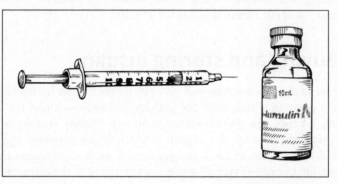

FIGURE 6-1:
An insulin syringe and vial of insulin.

Illustration by Kathryn Born, MA

Your syringe will also come with a needle. Needles can vary in length and diameter (also called *gauge*). Your healthcare provider can help you choose the optimal needle based on comfort and efficacy.

TIP

After you're done with your syringe, dispose of it properly as medical waste. Don't just throw it in your kitchen trash (ick) because it could poke someone carrying out the garbage or your garbage collector and spread disease. Instead, use a puncture-proof container like an old liquid detergent bottle at home or buy a convenient travel container for disposing of syringes when you're on the go.

REMEMBER

Fear of needles is a common concern among people starting insulin. You're not the only one who gets the heebie-jeebies when looking at a sharp needle. Don't keep these feelings inside. Tell someone on your healthcare team, such as a diabetes educator, nurse, or pharmacist, who can offer specific tips for overcoming this fear.

All about insulin pens

Most people who choose insulin pens do so for the convenience. You don't have to carry around a vial of insulin, and you don't have to draw up the insulin on the spot. You can also easily toss them in your bag or purse. However, insulin pens may be more expensive than using a syringe and vial, so do your homework.

Insulin pens (like the one shown in Figure 6-2) come in two styles: disposable (one-time use) and reusable (many times). Also, each pen is specially designed and manufactured to hold a particular type or mixture of insulin.

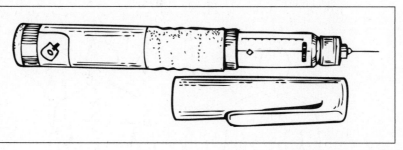

FIGURE 6-2:
An insulin pen.

Illustration by Kathryn Born, MA

Pen needles come in varying lengths and diameters, just like syringe needles. Screw on a new needle each time you inject insulin with your pen (needles can carry viruses or bacteria). Follow the instructions on your insulin pen to prime it. Then follow the dosing instructions from your healthcare provider, as well the instructions included with your pen.

Just like storing a vial of insulin, protect your insulin pen from extreme temperatures. You can keep pens you're currently using at room temperature and store unused pens in the refrigerator. Dispose of used needles in a safe container according to the package instructions.

Tips for injecting insulin

You don't just inject insulin anywhere you want on your body. That's not safe. Instead, there are techniques and tips for properly injecting insulin and making it as smooth and pain-free as possible. Ask your diabetes educator, nurse, or another provider for step-by-step instructions on injecting insulin.

Insulin is injected, using a syringe or pen, into the layer of fat that lies directly under your skin. The fancy name for this fat is *subcutaneous tissue*. Some of the best places to do that are your abdomen, thighs, and the backs of your upper arms. Your healthcare provider can instruct you on the best places to inject insulin and how to do it.

You can rotate the exact site of the injection so you don't get lumps or buildup of scar tissue. One technique is to think of the injection site as a 1-inch diameter circle. Choose a different, non-overlapping circle each time you inject and rotate within that part of your body, such as your abdomen. For site rotation techniques see Figure 6-3.

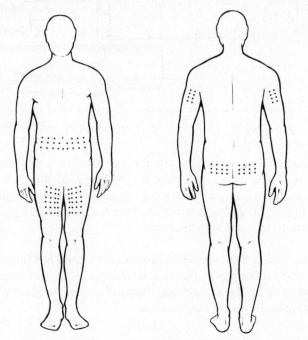

Courtesy of the American Diabetes Association

FIGURE 6-3:
Injection site rotation techniques.

TIP

Injecting insulin isn't easy for some people. Those with dexterity or vision problems, for example, may need a little extra help. There are lots of devices on the market that can help you overcome pain, anxiety, vision impairment, and dexterity challenges. Check out the latest issue of *Diabetes Forecast*'s annual consumer guide for details on injection aids or search the web for *injection aids* and look for highly rated and popular injection aids.

Insulin pumps

An insulin pump is another option for people with type 2 diabetes who need to give themselves multiple injections of insulin each day. People choose insulin pumps because they might help them better manage their blood glucose. Pumps can be convenient and can offer more flexibility to your insulin routine.

An *insulin pump* (shown in Figure 6-4) is a small device that you wear on your body that holds and delivers insulin. It's attached to a thin needle, called a *cannula*, that you insert under your skin. Some pumps are directly attached to the needle, and others are connected through tubing (called an *insertion set*) to deliver the insulin.

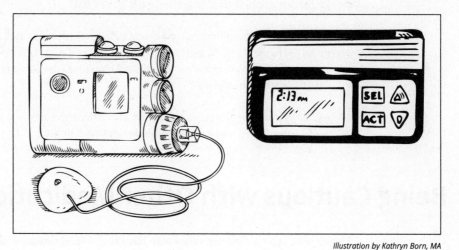

FIGURE 6-4:
An insulin pump with its insertion set.

Illustration by Kathryn Born, MA

TECHNICAL STUFF

Basal rate is the steady trickle of low levels of rapid-acting insulin in an insulin pump.

Most pumps deliver frequent, tiny doses of insulin at a steady background (basal) rate throughout the day and night and short bursts of insulin (bolus) before meals. You can program the pump to deliver insulin ahead of time, based on your expected needs. You can also push a button to deliver an extra bolus of insulin at mealtimes or snacks. This could also be used to treat episodes of high blood glucose.

TECHNICAL STUFF

An insulin pump on the market, called V-GO, is specifically used by people with type 2 diabetes. The pump is simple in that it attaches with a sticky patch to your skin and includes a built-in needle (no tubing required).

Most pumps fit inside a pump case that you wear on your waistband, bra, pocket, or similar spots that you find convenient. Your pump holds and dispenses your insulin, but that's not all. Pumps have a screen to display information and electronics to keep them running, and they can store data. Some pumps have special features like connecting wirelessly with blood glucose monitors or even integrating with a continuous glucose monitor (CGM).

CREATING AN ARTIFICIAL PANCREAS

You may have heard the term *artificial pancreas* and thought, "Wow, creepy!" or perhaps "Wow, cool!" Either way, artificial pancreases have been the dream of many for years — and they're finally approaching reality. Manufacturers have designed and are now testing devices that combine both an insulin pump and a CGM.

In 2016, the FDA approved the first type of artificial pancreas called a *hybrid closed-loop system*. A CGM monitors blood glucose every 5 minutes and automatically tells the pump how much insulin to dispense. Patients still have to tell the pump how much insulin to dispense at mealtimes.

Largely, the hybrid closed-loop system mimics what a pancreas does naturally in people without diabetes. That's how it got its name, the artificial pancreas.

Being Cautious with Other Medications

People with type 2 diabetes often also have high blood pressure and high cholesterol, so you may take medication for these conditions as well. High blood pressure and cholesterol increase your risk for cardiovascular disease, stroke, and other complications, so it's important to keep these in check. It's particularly important for people with diabetes because they are about two to three times more likely to die from heart disease than people without diabetes.

Eating healthier foods like those with less sodium or saturated fat, exercising more often, losing weight, and stopping smoking will help lower blood pressure and cholesterol. You may also need to take medication to achieve your goals.

Medication to lower blood pressure

Your body delivers blood and essential nutrients through its network of blood vessels. Blood pressure is the force at which blood pumps through your vessels. It's measured as a ratio of two numbers: *systolic blood pressure* (the pressure of blood in your vessels when your heart beats and pushes blood out) and *diastolic blood pressure* (the pressure in your vessels between heartbeats). Systolic is the first number; diastolic is the second number.

Your provider should measure your blood pressure at each visit. Most people with diabetes have a blood pressure goal of less than 140/90 mmHg.

Four classes of drugs are often used to lower blood pressure in people with diabetes including ACE inhibitors, angiotensin II receptor blockers (ARBs), thiazide-like diuretics, or dihydropyridine calcium channel blockers. Sometimes people will take more than one blood pressure medication to achieve their goals.

TIP

Remembering to take your medications can be difficult, especially if you take a lot of them every day. Pill organizers can help you organize your pills by day and time of day. You can buy them at a pharmacy or online. Noting that you've taken a medication by writing it down on a paper calendar or setting an alarm on your phone can also help. Put your medications in a hard-to-forget place like the kitchen table or next to your toothbrush.

Medication to treat cholesterol

High triglycerides, high LDL cholesterol (bad cholesterol), and low HDL cholesterol (good cholesterol) increase your risk of cardiovascular disease and stroke.

Your provider should measure these blood lipids, called a lipid profile, when you're first diagnosed with diabetes and then periodically thereafter. Statins, including atorvastatin (Lipitor) and simvastatin (Zocor), are medications that reduce the level of bad cholesterol and may increase good cholesterol. The American Diabetes Association recommends that most adults with diabetes take a statin. Other cholesterol-lowering drugs are also used in some patients with specific cardiovascular risks.

TECHNICAL
STUFF

LDL cholesterol stands for low-density lipoprotein; it's the "bad" cholesterol because it narrows and blocks arteries, which can lead to heart disease and stroke. Try to lower your LDL cholesterol. *HDL cholesterol* stands for high-density lipoprotein; it's the "good" cholesterol because it helps keep your blood vessels clear. Try to boost your HDL.

TIP

Eating healthy foods low in saturated fats, losing weight, exercising, and quitting smoking can have the beneficial effects of lowering LDL cholesterol and raising HDL cholesterol. It's a double bonus!

Aspirin and other medications

Ask your provider whether it makes sense for you to take a low dose of aspirin (81 mg) daily. People with diabetes who are 50 years old or older and who also have at least one additional risk factor for heart disease (such as high blood pressure, smoking, or high blood fats) may take a daily low-dose aspirin.

TIP

If you're overweight and struggling to lose those necessary pounds, you may consider asking your healthcare provider whether weight loss medications could help. Five weight loss medications are available for people with a body mass index (BMI) of more than 27 kg/m² and type 2 diabetes (or another medical condition).

They include orlistat (Alli, Xenical), lorcaserin (Belviq), phentermine/topiramate ER (Qsymia), Naltrexone/buproprion (Contrave), and liraglutide (Saxenda). All have common and more serious side effects. None of them should be used by pregnant women or those considering pregnancy.

TIP

BMI is a measurement of your weight (in kilograms) divided by height (in meters squared). It is used to tell whether you're underweight, normal weight, overweight, or obese. You can calculate your BMI at www.nhlbi.nih.gov/health/educational/lose_wt/BMI/bmicalc.htm (or just search online for *BMI calculator*).

Surgery for Type 2 Diabetes

Eating healthy foods, exercising, losing weight, and of course, taking necessary medications like pills or insulin are all proven strategies to manage your blood glucose and prevent complications. But now, some people with diabetes have another effective option: surgery.

Surgery to treat diabetes is called *metabolic surgery.* It is also sometimes called *bariatric surgery* or *weight-loss surgery.* The goal of metabolic surgery is to treat diabetes while helping patients lose weight and reduce the risk of cardiovascular disease. Some patients don't have to take diabetes medications anymore after surgery.

Several studies have shown that surgery can help people with type 2 diabetes improve their blood glucose and reduce their risk for cardiovascular disease. What's incredible is that these surgeries improve blood glucose in ways that extend beyond just losing weight. Scientists are still investigating this phenomenon.

Who is eligible for surgery? You must be a good candidate for surgery in order to get metabolic surgery, so ask your healthcare provider whether this might be a good option for you. For example, people with substance abuse problems or mental health conditions might not be the best candidates for surgery.

Then you and your doctor will consider your BMI and blood glucose control. The American Diabetes Association has very specific guidelines on who is an appropriate candidate for metabolic surgery. Recently, the Association recommended metabolic surgery for people with type 2 diabetes who are morbidly obese (BMI greater than 40 kg/m²) and in people with type 2 diabetes with uncontrolled blood glucose and a BMI between 35–39.9 kg/m². The Association also said that metabolic surgery can be considered in people with type 2 diabetes with a BMI of 30–34.9 kg/m² if their blood glucose is not adequately controlled.

Consider and weigh the adverse affects: Surgery is expensive and can cause long-term side effects such as a *dumping syndrome* (nausea, colic, and diarrhea), risk for depression, vitamin and mineral deficiencies, and other issues.

The four most commonly performed metabolic surgeries are: roux-en Y gastric bypass, vertical sleeve gastrectomy, laparoscopic adjustable gastric banding, and biliopancreatic diversion.

WARNING

Health insurance companies require different criteria for coverage of surgery, so do your homework. If you're considering metabolic surgery, call your insurance carrier to find out more about your coverage and limits.

3

Checking Blood Glucose and Reducing Complications

IN THIS PART . . .

Monitor your blood glucose and find out how the Rule of 15 can be used to treat low blood glucose.

Discover how your blood vessels affect your entire body — from your eyes to your feet — and find out how to keep them healthy to avoid complications.

Get familiar with health issues specific to women and men, including sexual wellness.

Chapter **7**

Checking Your Blood Glucose

Checking your blood glucose is essential for managing diabetes. It helps you gauge your body's reaction to medications, food, exercise, stress, sickness, and more. You'll use this information in your daily life, and you'll share this information with your healthcare provider to evaluate how things are going at checkups.

A blood glucose check is a snapshot of your blood glucose level that you can do anytime, anywhere. It's separate from the A1C test used in the doctor's office to diagnose diabetes or to measure your average blood glucose.

If you're newly diagnosed, checking your blood glucose might be the first skill you learn. It may seem foreign at first, but be patient. You'll get the hang of it. Checking blood glucose has never been easier or faster; we walk you through the steps in this chapter.

When and how often you check your blood glucose is highly individual. It depends on your goals, medications, and health. However, the American Diabetes Association has recommended guidelines, which we include in this chapter.

Checking your blood glucose also means doing something with that important information. We've got you covered. At the end of the chapter, we offer tips for tracking the data and explain what to do with it.

Why, When, and How to Check Your Blood Glucose Level

Your blood glucose level tells you about your body, and many factors can affect the numbers. If you're stressed or sick, or you forget to take your medication, your numbers may be high. If you don't eat enough or exercise for a long time, your numbers may be low. Strive to have your before-meal blood glucose number in the 80–130 mg/dL range and below 180 mg/dL 1–2 hours after meals.

REMEMBER

Knowing your numbers helps you feel better in the short term and helps you prevent complications down the road. This section explains the ins and outs of checking your blood glucose level.

Knowing when to check your glucose level

When you're first diagnosed with diabetes, you may feel like it's annoying to check your blood glucose. It's not uncommon for newbies to be overwhelmed or intimidated. The good news is that it gets easier with practice.

TIP

Talk with your doctor about how often and when to check your blood glucose. Before a meal or 2 hours after a meal are common times, but it's really up to you and your healthcare provider. The timing of the checks isn't set in stone. Instead, it's based on your goals, lifestyle, health, and medications.

Some people may need to check their blood glucose in the mornings or late at night because they tend to have high or low blood glucose at those times. If you're wondering how certain foods or types of exercise affect your blood glucose, you could check after you eat or work out.

If you use multiple daily injections of insulin, you'll need to check before and often after every meal to see how food affects your blood glucose. Check when you wake up to make sure your blood glucose is in your target range to start the day. Check before and after exercise to know whether you need to eat something to balance the calories you burned.

Occasionally you'll need to check your glucose levels at other times. If you're sick or recovering from an illness, your blood glucose may be high (above 180 mg/dL or your individual target) or low (below 70 mg/dL), so you'll need to keep an eye on it.

If you take oral medications or long-acting insulin, ask your healthcare provider when and how often to check your blood glucose. If you take multiple daily injections of insulin, you'll check more often, so ask about those specifics, too.

Checking your blood glucose in a snap

Blood isn't something most people think about or deal with very often. However, after you're diagnosed with diabetes, that changes. You have to prick your finger to check your blood glucose levels. In time, you'll be an expert and do it without even thinking about it. Some people are uncomfortable checking blood glucose in public, but there is no reason to be, and it can take as little as 15–20 seconds.

You use a blood glucose meter to check your glucose level (we cover glucose meters in the following section). Here are the steps to check your blood glucose:

1. **Wash and dry your hands.**
2. **Insert a test strip into your meter.**
3. **Use a lancing device to prick the side of your finger and draw a small sample of blood.**
4. **Hold your finger to the test strip.**
5. **Wait for the reading.**
6. **Once it displays, record the reading or use it to take action.**

Replace your lancet as necessary to keep the tip from getting dull and to make pricks more comfortable. (Find out more about lancets in the "Looking at lancets and test strips" section, later in the chapter.)

Eyeing your blood glucose targets

Together, you and your healthcare provider will figure out target ranges for blood glucose based on your goals. Targets are based on how long you've had diabetes, your age, complications, and other individual considerations.

The American Diabetes Association recommends these targets for most non-pregnant adults:

>> **A1C:** Less than 7

>> **Before a meal:** 80–130 mg/dL

>> **After a meal (1–2 hours after beginning a meal):** Less than 180 mg/dL

However, different targets may be better for certain individuals. If you're a senior, your doctor may say you don't need to worry as much about keeping blood glucose in that tight range. If you're pregnant, you'll have different goals so you can keep the baby as healthy as can be (see more in Chapter 9).

Blood Glucose Meters and Accessories

Use a small, portable device called a *blood glucose meter* to measure the amount of glucose in your blood.

TIP

Think about your needs and do some research before you select a meter. For example, some meters may benefit people with limited vision or dexterity issues, or you may want the latest technology. Test strips go hand-in-hand with meters, so consider them as well. A meter that may be very low cost or free through a promotion may use more expensive test strips, and cost a lot in the long run. Select among certain meters based on your health insurance coverage. We give you an overview of meters, their features, and test strips in this section.

Checking out types of meters

Blood glucose meters have come a long way since they were first invented, but they all have the same basic parts.

Each device has a small slot where you insert a test strip. You take your test strip out of its container (a vial or package) and pop it in the slot. You prick your finger with a lancet to produce a drop of blood, and the test strip has chemicals that react with your blood glucose to give a reading.

You view the results of your blood test on a digital screen. A reading will appear as number (say, 100), followed by mg/dL (milligrams per deciliter). The number represents the amount of glucose in your blood.

Today you can find dozens of meters with all sorts of bells and whistles. But before you start drooling over all the latest features, you have to choose the type of device that works best for you. Luckily, they fall into two main categories: standard blood glucose meters and continuous glucose meters.

Standard blood glucose meters

A standard blood glucose meter reads your blood glucose in one moment. It's just a snapshot. Prick, drop, and — voilà! — there it is. A standard blood glucose meter is what almost everyone with diabetes uses to check their blood glucose.

Continuous glucose meters

A continuous glucose meter (CGM) takes continuous readings of glucose levels in real time, rather than providing a snapshot. You wear the device all the time, although you change the sensor every few days depending on the brand and type.

A CGM has three parts: sensor, transmitter, and receiver.

You insert the sensor under your skin to monitor your interstitial fluid, which cor-relates to blood glucose. The sensor readings are wirelessly transmitted to a hand-held receiver. The receiver displays blood glucose levels in real time and includes past readings.

The beauty and elegance of a CGM is that you can see blood glucose trends over time — whether you're trending up or down. The receiver displays graphs and arrows pointing up or down.

TIP

Use these trends to make decisions about insulin or food. A CGM can also alert you to a high or low. You may choose to share these real-time readings with your doctor or family members so they can help monitor your health. Some CGMs are designed to work with meters and insulin pumps to streamline use.

TIP

Check with your insurance provider about coverage for CGMs, which are more likely to be covered for people who have type 1 diabetes.

Being aware of meter accuracy

The U.S. Food and Drug Administration (FDA) has established guidelines regarding the accuracy of blood glucose meters. Because millions of people use and rely on these devices, it's important that they give the most accurate readings possible.

Manufacturers are now required to clearly state the accuracy of their meters on the outside of boxes and test strips. These are shown as percentages (95 percent accuracy, for example). This data will help you buy a better, more accurate meter.

REMEMBER

A more accurate meter will lead you to make correct decisions about controlling your diabetes. If a meter shows inaccurate results, you may take an incorrect action that could have serious consequences. Bottom line: Pay attention to meter accuracy.

TIP

The FDA has these recommendations for testing your meter's performance:

>> Some meters use a liquid control solution (containing a known amount of glucose). Use the control solution in place of a blood sample to see whether the results match the range listed on your test strips. An unusual number could mean you have a problem with your meter or your test strips.

>> Your meter also runs its own electronic check each time it's turned on so keep an eye out for error codes and consult your instructions if you see one.

>> Bring your meter with you for your next checkup. Show your provider your technique and measure your meter's reading with a laboratory blood test.

Considering a multitude of meter features

As technology advances, so do the features you can find in blood glucose meters. You can find basic meters that do nothing more than measure your glucose level and save your numbers. On the other end of the spectrum, you can find meters that calculate your mealtime insulin dose, have a backlit screen for testing in the dark, and work with your smartphone. How fancy a meter you want is up to you.

The following lists include some options to consider if you have special circumstances.

If you have vision problems:

>> A **high-contrast screen** makes readings easier to see.

>> **Audio features** such as a talking meter may help.

>> A **backlight** could make readings easier to see, especially at night.

>> **Port lights** help you insert test strips and take readings at night.

If dexterity is a challenge:

>> **Larger meters** are easier to grip.

>> **Larger test strips** with easy-to-grasp containers could help.

If you like using the latest technology, most meters allow you to download readings that detail the date, time, result, and other information to a software program on your computer or other device. Some meters wirelessly transmit readings to your smartphone or the cloud (using Wi-Fi or Bluetooth).

In addition to measuring your glucose level, some meters measure blood pressure or ketones. (We explain the importance of these measures in Chapter 8.)

Other meters offer access to certified diabetes educators (CDEs) and advice. A meter that includes a *bolus calculator* (a feature that tells you how much insulin is needed at mealtime) is a plus for people on intensive insulin therapy. Finally, you may want a meter that lets you test in other areas of your body, such as your arms or thighs, if you get calluses on your fingertips that make them hard to prick.

Minding money matters

Because blood glucose meters offer many different features and designs, they're available at a wide range of price points. You're guaranteed to find one that fits your budget.

Devices range in cost from $10 or so to $150. However, don't think you have to spend a bundle on a blood glucose meter. You can buy a decent one for around $20.

Your healthcare provider will give you a prescription for the meter, test strips, and lancets. These tools are also available over the counter. However, having prescriptions for your health insurance or Medicare can help cover the costs.

TIP

Do your homework. Your health insurance or Medicare may cover only certain meters and test strips. What if your healthcare provider prescribes a meter that isn't covered? Ask him to write a letter to your health insurer to obtain coverage, or ask him whether you can change meters and use one that is covered by your insurance.

Medicare Part B covers the cost of meters, test strips, lancet devices, and lancets. You can buy testing supplies through Medicare's National Mail-Order Program for delivery to your home or from any local pharmacy or store that's enrolled with Medicare.

Not only do you have to consider the meter's cost, but you also have to think about how much the test strips will cost you on a monthly or yearly basis. In the long run, your meter's test strips will cost you much more than the meter itself.

TIP

If you don't have insurance or you're having trouble affording your test strips, you have some options. Some strip manufacturers offer assistance programs, and some governmental and local groups may offer discounted supplies. Ask your healthcare provider or pharmacist about these programs.

You might also consider switching to generic, instead of brand name, meter and strips, such as those sold by CVS, Rite Aid, Target, Walgreens, and Walmart.

Every year, the American Diabetes Association's magazine, *Diabetes Forecast*, publishes a consumer guide to blood glucose meters and other products. You can read the consumer guide with a print subscription or access it online at www.diabetesforecast.org.

Looking at lancets and test strips

Blood glucose meters need two accessories in order to work: lancets and test strips.

A *lancet* is a device that pricks the skin to get a small blood sample. Lancets are available in many different brands and types. Some devices have preloaded lancets so you never have to touch them. Some allow you to get a sample with just one click, so it's easy and fast. Others have settings for how deep the lancet goes based on what feels better to you.

WARNING

Don't share or reuse lancets — they're only sterile the first time.

After you've drawn a drop of blood, you apply it to a test strip. These disposable strips absorb your blood and feed it into the blood glucose meter. You use a new one every time you take a sample.

Your test strips are made to work with your meter. You'll need to buy the brand name or generic test strip that fits. They'll come in a box with one or two vials of test strips.

Keeping Track of Data

Checking blood glucose is the best way to monitor your diabetes. However, it's not just an important reading. Your health depends on how you use that data to take better care of yourself.

An important step is writing down or downloading readings so you can see how your daily activities affect your blood glucose. In addition to the reading, keep track of the date and time, as well as details like what you ate or how long you exercised.

Choosing a tracking method that works for you

The way in which you record your data is up to you. Paper logbooks, spreadsheets, and apps are all good options.

You may like to write readings down on a piece of paper or in a logbook. Recording the results with pen and paper can help you learn about your condition and interpret the readings.

Or you may like the convenience of having your readings stored in your meter. Meters can store hundreds of readings, although eventually you'll need to download them onto a computer to free up more memory. Downloading them and viewing them in a software program or spreadsheet helps you see the big picture.

You can use a meter or CGM that automatically uploads results to the cloud over Wi-Fi or Bluetooth so you don't have to physically plug your meter into a computer. You can then view these readings in a software program or app at your convenience.

There is no shortage of apps to help you track your blood glucose data. Search iTunes or Google Play for apps that might work for you. New ones are added all the time.

TIP

Make sure you bring your blood glucose readings with you when you visit your doctor or diabetes educator. Beforehand, ask your provider how she likes to look at readings in the office. Your provider may prefer a paper printout, or she may have a computer and software to download readings from your meter on site.

Putting the numbers to use

The most important part of gathering data is putting it to work. The best way to do this is to talk with your healthcare provider. Together, you'll come up with goals and targets for your blood glucose. You'll take your readings to your check-ups and talk about why there were highs and lows — and what to do about them. As you get the hang of it, you may use the readings to learn when you need to add a snack to your meal plan or get more exercise during the day, for example.

How you use your readings also depends on how often you check your glucose level. If you check once a day, that reading might give you a general idea about how your medications are working. Think big picture. If you check three times a day, you might learn when you need to eat less (or different types of food), exercise more, or destress. Focus on making small changes.

Keeping a record is an individual action, but it's important for everyone with diabetes. It's universal. Whether you check your blood glucose once a day or seven times a day, you'll see trends over time about how different things like food, exercise, oral medications, or insulin affect your blood glucose. The goal is to tweak those things to reach a balance so most of your readings are in your target ranges. You'll find out more specifics about this in Part 4 on food and exercise.

Without data, you just have guesses. It doesn't matter whether a reading is in range. The most important thing is to record it and discuss it with your healthcare provider.

It's natural to feel disappointed if your reading isn't what you expected. Try not to fall into this mind-set. It's not helpful to view readings as "good" or "bad." They're just data giving you more information about your body and your diabetes.

Putting your data to work also means reducing the risk of complications like extremely high blood glucose (also called *hyperglycemia*), which can make you tired and thirsty or blur your vision, and extremely low blood glucose (or *hypoglycemia*), which can make you hungry, make you irritable, or even make you pass out. Very high blood glucose can eventually lead to or worsen diabetes complications, and both high and low blood glucose levels can be very dangerous if untreated. (Read more about high and low blood glucose in the next chapter.)

Chapter **8**

Keeping Complications in Check

You can live a long, healthy life with diabetes. The key to success is keeping your blood glucose on target. Why? High or low blood glucose isn't good for your body.

In the short term, high blood glucose can make you feel thirsty, tired, and out of sorts. And low blood glucose can cause dizziness, confusion, and inability to concentrate. Left untreated, either condition can be dangerous or even fatal.

In the long term, chronically high blood glucose damages your blood vessels, causing them to swell, become blocked, or leak. This can happen all over your body — in your heart, brain, eyes, kidneys, and legs. Healthy blood vessels are the secret to a healthy body.

High blood glucose can also damage your nerves, causing pain or numbness in your feet and problems with *autonomic body systems* (the body's functions that happen without your thinking about them, like your digestive and cardiovascular systems).

However, despite your best efforts, you'll probably have very high or low readings at some point, particularly if you use insulin (see Chapter 7 for more about measuring your blood glucose level). It's part of having diabetes. But the goal should be for most of your readings to fall within the ranges your healthcare provider recommends for you.

REMEMBER

The best way to avoid wide swings in your blood glucose level is by eating healthy meals and taking your medications on a regular schedule.

In this chapter, you find out more about complications and how to prevent them. You can take steps now to head off complications so you feel good tomorrow and when you're 92.

Looking Out for Lows

If you have a blood glucose reading below 70 mg/dL, it's called *hypoglycemia*, or low blood glucose. This number is just a guideline, so make sure you discuss lows with your doctor. You need to know what is low for you so you can take action at the right time and with the right tools.

Lows can happen to people who use insulin or certain oral medications.

Low blood glucose is dangerous because you can get dizzy or pass out. You could hit your head or drive off the side of the road. In the most serious cases, hypoglycemia can cause seizures, coma, and death.

In the following sections, we outline the warning signs that alert you that you're having a low, and we tell you how to bring your blood glucose level up quickly.

Knowing the warning signs of lows

You may notice when you're having a low because you feel sweaty, confused, or just not right. A low may come on gradually, so you pick up on these symptoms. Or it may come on suddenly, so you don't feel that different.

Here are common signs of low blood glucose:

>> Shaking

>> Nervousness or anxiety

>> Sweating, chills, and clamminess

- » Irritability

- » Color draining from the skin

- » Hunger and nausea

- » Rapid heartbeat

- » Weakness, fatigue, and sleepiness

- » Headache

- » Tingling or numbness in the lips or tongue

- » Nightmares or crying out during sleep

- » Lightheadedness, dizziness, or confusion

- » Difficulty seeing or blurry vision

- » Unusual behavior such as clumsiness or slurring of words

- » Anger, sadness, and/or stubbornness

Some signs of *severely* low blood glucose include the following:

- » Seizures

- » Unconsciousness

People usually experience signs of lows, but the signs are a little different for each person. Make a point to tell your spouse, family, or friends about the signs of low blood glucose so they can look out for them and help you if the time comes. (We explain how to treat lows in the following section.)

REMEMBER

If you think you're low, check your blood glucose. Checking your blood glucose is the only way to know for sure whether you're low (see Chapter 7).

TIP

Often people with diabetes can't tell when they're low, particularly when they've had diabetes for a long time. *Hypoglycemia unawareness* is a fancy term for when you can't feel lows. Talk to your doctor if you suspect you might have this condition.

Treating lows with the Rule of 15

After you test your blood glucose to confirm that you're low, then treat yourself right away. The goal is to raise your blood glucose. You can do this simply by eating or drinking.

Quickly and effectively raise your blood glucose using fast-acting carbohydrates, without fat or protein mixed in, which include the following:

>> Four glucose tablets

>> Four ounces of fruit juice or soda (not diet)

>> Eight ounces of nonfat or 1 percent milk

>> Two tablespoons of raisins

>> Glucose gels, or liquids (more on these coming up)

Each of these foods has 15 grams of carbohydrates and is suitable for use with the Rule of 15.

What the heck is the Rule of 15? It's an easy trick for treating lows. But before you use the Rule of 15, ask your doctor whether it's right for you. Your doctor will tell you what to do if you shouldn't use the Rule of 15 for some reason.

Here are the five steps for the Rule of 15:

1. **Test your blood glucose (see Chapter 7).**

2. **If your blood glucose is below 70 mg/dL, eat or drink something containing 15–20 grams of carbohydrates.**

3. **Wait 15 minutes.**

4. **Test again. If your level is still below 70 mg/dL, eat or drink another 15 grams of carbohydrates.**

5. **Repeat until normal.**

When using the Rule of 15, consider eating a snack if your planned meal is an hour or more away.

If you can't always have fruit juice, milk, or raisins available to treat your lows, you can buy tablets, gels, and liquids that come prepackaged as exactly 15 grams of carbohydrates. They're made just for people with diabetes. They work fast and are easy to have on hand. Pop them in your purse, car, or desk drawer so you have them when you need them. If you don't have a supply on hand, drink a glass of milk or juice.

Generic or store-brand glucose products may be cheaper than brand-name versions, so shop around.

Having glucagon available

It's rare, but sometimes people become so low that they pass out and can't treat themselves. In this emergency, someone else must give them an injection of glucagon.

What's glucagon? It's a hormone that your body makes to raise blood glucose. But it's also a medication in a portable kit for emergencies. The kit has a vial of powder and a syringe of saline that someone mixes together and injects, following the instructions.

Not everyone needs a glucagon kit, so ask your healthcare provider if you're concerned. He can write a prescription for one if he thinks you might be at risk for lows. Teach family members and co-workers how to use the kit, and tell them to call 911 if they have any concerns.

Heading Off Highs

Hyperglycemia, or high blood glucose, describes glucose levels that are higher than normal.

High blood glucose can make you feel thirsty, out of sorts, or tired. It can blur your vision, cause itchy skin, or make you pee a lot. The signs of high blood glucose are slower to develop and more likely to be missed for long periods of time than the signs of low blood glucose.

TIP

The *dawn phenomenon* is when you get a high blood glucose reading early in the morning, generally between 4 a.m. and 6 a.m. It's quite common, and it happens naturally because of hormones. If you suspect the dawn phenomenon is giving you high readings, ask your healthcare provider how to manage it.

Over time, high blood glucose can damage blood vessels in your body, leading to heart disease, stroke, blindness, and kidney failure. You find out more on these specific complications later in the chapter.

Eating too much, forgetting to take your medications, or getting sick can cause highs. Taking a walk is a good way to lower blood glucose in the short term.

For the long term, ask your healthcare provider how you should manage high blood glucose. You might need to eat healthier foods, exercise more, or switch your medications.

In the following sections, we describe two serious conditions that can arise from hyperglycemia.

Diabetic ketoacidosis

Diabetic ketoacidosis (DKA) occurs when you have consistent, extremely high blood glucose of 250 mg/dL or above. It happens more often in people with type 1 diabetes than in people with type 2 diabetes.

DKA usually happens when people are sick and their bodies make ketones in their blood and urine that build up and become toxic. It's a dangerous situation that can cause breathing difficulties, shock, pneumonia, seizures, coma, and even death.

Ketones are chemicals that are produced when the body burns fat instead of glucose for energy. This process occurs when the body doesn't have enough insulin for the amount of glucose it needs to use.

Luckily, you can test for ketones using a simple test strip from the pharmacy. Generally, you check for ketones by dipping a test strip into your urine stream, or you pee into a cup and dip a strip, and then you get a reading. However, follow the specific instructions that come with the test strips. Treating hyperglycemia in a timely fashion will usually prevent ketoacidosis when ketones are first present.

Some blood glucose meters also measure ketones, so check whether your meter has that option.

The warning signs of DKA include the following:

>> Blood glucose of 250 mg/dL or above

>> Nausea or vomiting

>> Fruity breath odor

>> Rapid breathing

>> Flushed sensation

>> Weakness

>> Drowsiness

>> Intense thirst

>> Dry mouth

>> Need to urinate frequently

>> Lack of appetite

>> Stomach pains

Ask your healthcare provider about if and when you should check for ketones. She may recommend checking every 4–6 hours if you're sick or if you get a blood glucose reading above 240 mg/dL. She may also want you to call if you have ketones so she can give you further instructions.

Hyperosmolar hyperglycemic syndrome

Hyperosmolar hyperglycemic syndrome (HHS) is caused by extremely high blood glucose. It can be brought on by other conditions like not taking enough medication, infections, heart attack, or stroke. It usually happens over time. HHS can cause severe dehydration, seizures, coma, and even death.

You can develop HHS if you have high blood glucose and don't drink enough fluids. People who are elderly and those who are in the hospital or a nursing home are at higher risk for HHS.

It can take days or weeks for HHS to develop, so always drink plenty of fluids — particularly when you're sick.

Here are the warning signs that you may be developing HHS:

>> Blood glucose of 600 mg/dL or higher

>> Dry, parched mouth

>> Extreme thirst (although this symptom may gradually disappear)

>> Warm, dry skin with no sweat

>> High fever

>> Sleepiness or confusion

TIP

For caregivers: If your parent or an elderly relative with type 2 diabetes is in a nursing home or hospital, make sure drinking water is available, and encourage your loved one to drink water often. Some older people don't recognize when they're thirsty, so they may need extra reminders.

Maintaining a Healthy Heart and Brain

Keeping both your heart and brain healthy is important. People with diabetes are about two to three times more likely to die from heart disease than people without diabetes.

Heart disease leads to chest pain, heart attacks, and heart failure. Strokes, which are caused by an interruption of blood flow to your brain, lead to difficulty speaking or walking or numbness in your face, arms, or legs. Both are cardiovascular complications, which are caused by damaged blood vessels.

Your blood vessels deliver blood, oxygen, and nutrients to your body, so it's critical that you keep them healthy. Healthy vessels reduce the risk of heart disease and stroke. Here are some ways to keep your blood vessels healthy:

» Keep your blood pressure in a healthy range.

» Keep your blood glucose on target.

» Quit smoking or don't start.

» Eat wholesome, nutritious foods low in saturated fat, cholesterol, and sodium.

» Lose weight.

» Exercise regularly.

» Take recommended medications for blood pressure, cholesterol, and blood glucose.

» Know the signs of heart disease and stroke.

TIP

Sleep apnea is the medical term for when your breathing stops and starts repeatedly during sleep. It is more common in people with diabetes and people who are overweight. It also increases your risk of cardiovascular disease. Talk to your healthcare provider about sleep apnea so you can get treatment if you need it.

The following sections give you an overview of complications that may develop in your cardiovascular system and brain if you don't control your diabetes.

Hardening of your arteries

Atherosclerosis is the term for hardening of the blood vessels called arteries. Hardening can happen with a buildup of fat and cholesterol that stops blood flow. It can occur in arteries supplying your heart, brain, and other organs.

You may sometimes hear the term *metabolic syndrome* (or *cardiometabolic syndrome*) when you hear about diabetes and heart disease. Metabolic syndrome is a collection of various risk factors that tend to group together (obesity, high blood glucose, hypertension, high blood fat levels) and can lead to heart disease.

Heart attacks

A heart attack occurs when a blood clot forms in an artery and stops blood flow to your heart. Part of the heart muscle dies or is damaged during a heart attack.

Know the signs of a heart attack:

>> Discomfort or pain in your chest, arms, back, jaw, neck, or stomach (yes, any one of these places)

>> Shortness of breath

>> Sweating

>> Indigestion or nausea

>> Lightheadedness

>> Fatigue

Call 911 immediately if you suspect you or someone else is having a heart attack.

Strokes

The most common type of stroke, an *ischemic stroke*, occurs when a blood vessel gets clogged and stops blood flow to your brain, usually because of a blood clot. Another type of stroke, called a *hemorrhagic stroke*, occurs when a blood vessel leaks or breaks. During a stroke, brain cells die because they don't have enough blood or oxygen.

The signs of a stroke include numbness in the face, arm, or leg (especially on just one side instead of both). Confusion, severe headaches, or difficulty speaking, seeing, or walking are also signs of a stroke. The American Stroke Association suggests the acronym *FAST* to remind you of these symptoms: *F* for face drooping, *A* for arm weakness, *S* for speech difficulty, *T* for time to call 911.

Call 911 immediately if you suspect you or someone else is having a stroke.

Feeling Good in Your Skin

You may not believe it, but your skin is affected by diabetes. People with diabetes are more likely to have itchy skin, which can be caused by infections, dryness, or poor circulation. They're also more likely to have bacterial and fungal infections, which can be exacerbated by high blood glucose.

Dry skin can happen anywhere, but it may be common on your lower legs if you have poor circulation. Moisturize often, limit bathing time or frequency in the winter, and use mild soaps to prevent dry skin.

Common bacterial infections include sties, boils, and infections around nails. Prevent infections by keeping your blood glucose on target and keeping an eye out for any hot, swollen, or painful areas of your skin. Antibiotics can treat infections, so see your healthcare provider if you think you have an infection.

Common fungal infections include rashes in warm, moist areas of the body, such as between fingers and toes, under breasts, around the groin, and in the armpits. They're the same infections everyone else gets, like jock itch, athlete's foot, and vaginal infections. Topical creams can treat fungal infections, so ask your doctor for recommendations.

TIP

Most skin problems can be prevented or treated easily. Here are some strategies for keeping your skin feeling good:

>> Keep your blood glucose on target.

>> Avoid hot baths and showers or limit them if humidity is low, like during the winter.

>> Make sure skin is clean and dry.

>> Prevent dry skin by moisturizing, especially when it's cold.

>> Use mild soaps and shampoos.

>> Don't use feminine sprays.

>> Use a humidifier during cold, dry winter months.

>> Wear sunscreen and put on a hat if you're in the sun.

>> Drink plenty of water.

>> Treat cuts immediately by washing with soap and water and covering with sterile gauze.

>> See your doctor immediately if you get a major cut, burn, or infection.

>> Visit a dermatologist if you have concerns about your skin.

Keeping Your Mouth in Tip-Top Shape

Good tooth and gum habits will keep your mouth clean and prevent complications. Just as your skin is more prone to infection when you have diabetes, your gums may be more prone to infection, too. Gum disease is more common in people with diabetes.

High blood glucose can create a breeding ground for infections in your mouth, which is one more reason to keep your blood glucose on target. You should brush and floss regularly, as well as see a dentist for cleanings, exams, and early detection of gum disease. Tell your dentist and hygienist that you have type 2 diabetes.

Here are some oral hygiene hints:

>> Brush for 2 minutes a day twice a day with an anti-gingivitis toothpaste approved by the American Dental Association.

>> See your dentist every 6 months (more often, if needed).

>> Look for signs of gum disease and tell your dentist if you have red, puffy, sore, or bloody gums.

>> Tell your dentist if you notice your gums are pulling away from your teeth, your bite changes, or your breath is always bad.

Focusing on Your Eyes

Vision is one of the most important senses, so you need to pay special attention to your eyes when you have diabetes. You've heard this before, but healthy blood vessels are the key. When blood vessels in the eyes swell or rupture, they can cause vision problems and blindness.

Eye disease is pretty common in people with diabetes. Up to 40 percent of people with diabetes develop some degree of damage to the tiny blood vessels in the eye (*retinopathy*) at some point in their lives, and diabetic retinopathy is the leading cause of blindness among working-age adults in the United States.

How is your eye designed to help you see clearly? Let's start from the outside of your eyeball and work back in toward your skull.

Your eyeball has a cornea, which is a thin, clear tissue. The cornea allows light in and helps focus light to the back of the eye. Behind the cornea is your pupil, which is the dark spot that gets smaller when it's really sunny and bigger when it's really dark. It's in the center of your iris, which is the colored part of your eye that allows light inside.

Now, behind all that is your lens, which focuses to sharpen objects using muscles. Your retina is nerve tissue that takes the stuff you see and packages it into nerve impulses that travel through the optic nerve to your brain. Your retina has specialized cells to sense light (rods and cones), as well as lots of blood vessels to support those cells.

REMEMBER

Keep your blood glucose on target to prevent eye problems. Studies show that lowering blood glucose can substantially improve eye health in people with diabetes.

You can also take care of your eyes by getting regular exams from an eye specialist such as an optometrist or ophthalmologist. An eye exam gives the doctor an up-close look at the inner workings of your eyeballs for any signs of damage. You should have an eye exam when you're diagnosed with type 2 diabetes and then every 1–2 years after that.

Here are the key ways to ensure healthy eyes and good vision:

» Keep your blood glucose on target.

» Lower your blood pressure by eating healthy foods, exercising, or taking medications.

» Get a dilated eye exam every 1–2 years.

» Pay attention to changes in your vision such as blurriness, shadows, or difficulty seeing, and see a specialist if you have concerns.

The good news is that 90 percent of sight-threatening vision problems can be treated if they're caught early. Getting a dilated eye exam from an eye specialist is the best way to detect these early changes.

WARNING

People with diabetes are at an increased risk for cataracts and glaucoma, which can also be treated, especially if caught early. *Cataracts* are opaque, cloudy areas on the lens of the eye that can block vision. They're treated with a surgery in which the damaged lens is removed and an artificial lens is placed in the eye. *Glaucoma* is a condition in which the pressure inside the eye is higher than it should be. Glaucoma can damage the optic nerve and lead to blindness if not treated. Treatment includes eye drops and laser surgery.

Putting Your Best Foot Forward

People with diabetes may experience problems with their feet and lower legs. These problems arise when your blood vessels aren't healthy. You may also encounter problems with the nerves in your legs and feet. Good foot care is important because diabetes is the leading cause of amputation in adults, and amputation can be prevented in most cases by detecting and treating problems early.

The following sections explain how to take care of your extremities so small problems don't develop into more serious ones.

Getting a leg up on caring for your lower extremities

Keeping your blood glucose on target is the best way to keep your blood vessels healthy in your legs and feet and to protect your nerves (see the earlier section "Maintaining a Healthy Heart and Brain" for more about this). Controlling blood pressure is also very important. Exercise regularly and quit smoking to improve circulation in your legs and feet.

Because skin infections are more common in people with diabetes and often occur on the feet, preventing and treating foot problems is essential.

Protect your feet from calluses by wearing shoes that fit well. Buy comfortable shoes with low heels or thick soles to cushion your feet. If you get a callous, don't try to remove it on your own, but instead see your doctor or nurse so it's removed properly and doesn't cause an infection.

Protect your feet from *ulcers,* which are sores or holes in the skin on the bottom or sides of your feet. Treat cuts and blisters immediately and see a doctor if you have any concerns. Visually check your feet regularly for any signs of infection because damage to your nerves could affect *how much* you feel pain.

You should also get an annual foot exam from your healthcare provider in which he checks the sensation, blood flow, and bone structure of your feet. It may sound funny, but take off your socks and shoes when you get to your checkup. That way, you'll both remember to check out your feet.

Here's a checklist that can help you keep your feet and legs healthy:

>> Check both of your feet every day by comparing them and looking for cuts, blisters, ingrown toenails, or any other changes.

TIP

If you're elderly and can't bend over or see well, use a mirror or ask a relative for help inspecting your feet.

>> Keep your toenails trimmed or see a podiatrist for trimming if you can't do it yourself.

>> Get an annual foot exam.

>> Keep your blood glucose on target.

>> Wear comfortable socks and shoes that fit well.

>> Quit smoking and exercise regularly to improve circulation.

>> Talk to your doctor if you suspect peripheral artery disease (PAD; see the following section).

TIP

You'll definitely see socks specifically marketed and sold as "diabetes socks." These come as either over-the-counter socks that you can buy anywhere or prescription "compression" socks that your provider will prescribe to purchase online or at a medical supply store. These socks may have diabetes-specific features such as light to high compression (to reduce swelling) and antibacterial properties such as moisture-wicking fabric (to keep feet dry and prevent infections). Sometimes these socks don't have seams, which helps to prevent rubbing, irritation, and sores from developing. You don't *need* to buy "diabetes socks" unless your provider recommends it.

REMEMBER

Amputation can be a risk for people with diabetes. People with diabetes are at least 10 times more likely to have a lower-extremity amputation than people without diabetes. And in most of those cases, the amputation occurred because of a preexisting foot ulcer (an open sore or wound).

Why does this happen to people with diabetes? It's a combination of factors. People with diabetes may have nerve damage that prevents them from feeling sores and cuts that other people may notice (see more on neuropathy in the following section). Circulation and swelling problems can reduce blood flow, which can slow healing of these wounds. High blood glucose can prevent the body from fighting off infection.

However, you can prevent this by following the checklist earlier in this section, including lowering your blood glucose, inspecting your feet daily for sores, and getting an annual foot exam.

Peripheral artery disease

Peripheral artery disease (PAD) happens when blood vessels to the periphery (such as your legs) get clogged and limit blood flow. The condition can be painful, causing leg cramps and difficulty walking. It may also lead to more infections in your legs or feet because circulation is limited.

Your healthcare provider can diagnose PAD using a test called the ankle-brachial index, which measures the blood pressure in your arm compared to your ankle. If you're diagnosed with PAD, you'll want to find out about treatments such as exercise routines that start very slowly.

Healthy Nerves All Over Your Body

Your nerves form an amazing network that extends from your brain all the way down to your toes. Your nerves affect everything from how you grasp a pen in your hand to how you digest your food. If your nerves aren't healthy, the rest of your body won't be healthy.

There are two main types of *neuropathy* (nerve damage). One is called *peripheral neuropathy,* and it affects nerves in places like your hands, feet, and legs. The other is called *autonomic neuropathy,* and it affects nerves that control your heart rate, blood pressure, sweating, urination, bowel movements, digestion, and other functions that take place in your body without your thinking about them.

Keeping your blood glucose under control will help keep your nerves healthy and ease symptoms. We explain each type of neuropathy and the symptoms in the following sections.

Nerves that sense things

Peripheral neuropathy — nerve damage to your hands, feet, and legs — is the most common type of neuropathy. The damage can lead to numbness, tingling, or prickling sensations; shooting or stabbing pain; a sensation of bugs crawling on your skin or walking on a strange surface; or a complete loss of feeling.

A complete loss of feeling can be problematic because you may not be able to feel pain, heat, or cold in your feet, which means you may not notice infections or other pain you would normally sense. Wear water footwear when wading in water and wear shoes when walking on hot pavement or sand so you don't get a cut or burn your feet. Check your feet visually *every day* for cuts and sores. We can't stress enough how important this is.

TIP

Your healthcare provider can check for nerve function using vibrations or touch during your yearly exam.

Medications such as antidepressants and topical creams can ease neuropathy, so talk to your doctor if you're experiencing pain or other symptoms.

Nerves that automatically do things

Autonomic neuropathy — nerve damage to involuntary body functions such as digestion, urination, or the function of your heart — can cause problems, too.

One form is called gastroparesis, which can cause heartburn, nausea, or lack of appetite. Diabetes is the most common known cause of gastroparesis, according to the National Institute of Diabetes and Digestive and Kidney Diseases. Gastroparesis may also impede your best efforts to control your blood glucose because it causes a spike in blood glucose after eating. Nerve damage could cause diarrhea or constipation. Nevertheless, keeping your blood glucose in your target range is the best way to avoid damage to the nerves in your intestine and throughout your body.

Nerve damage can also affect your bladder's ability to fully empty or other urination problems. This could, in turn, increase your risk for urinary tract infections. Autonomic neuropathy could affect your sexual organs, increasing your risk for erectile dysfunction and ejaculation problems for men and vaginal dryness and difficulty achieving orgasm for women (see more about sexual health later in the chapter). Although these aren't fun topics to talk about, they're important to bring up with your healthcare provider.

Taking Care of Your Kidneys

Your kidneys filter waste out of your blood, and even though you may never think about them, they do essential work every day. The best way to take care of your kidneys is to keep your blood vessels healthy.

You can keep your kidney blood vessels healthy by keeping your blood glucose on target and lowering your blood pressure. Lower your blood pressure by eating healthy foods low in sodium, exercising, or taking medications.

A combination of high blood glucose and high blood pressure causes your kidneys to leak a protein called *albumin*, which makes your ankles and other parts of your body swell. That can be the first sign of kidney disease. If not treated, your kidneys may eventually become so damaged that they don't filter your blood anymore. Some people then need to go on dialysis to filter out waste or get a kidney transplant.

TECHNICAL STUFF

Dialysis is a medical procedure in which your blood is taken out through a needle, filtered by a machine outside your body, and then returned to your body through a separate needle. You go to a hospital or dialysis center to have the procedure, which usually takes a few hours and is done three times a week. You can also have dialysis in your home.

Take medications for blood glucose and blood pressure to prevent and treat kidney disease. Also, make sure you have yearly tests of both your urine and blood to determine whether you have signs of kidney disease.

There are two key markers for kidney disease: urine albumin and estimated glomerular filtration rate (eGFR). Too much protein in your urine (albumin) is a sign of kidney disease. Too much waste product in your blood (creatinine), measured through an eGFR blood test, is also a sign of kidney disease.

Coping with Burnout, Stress, and Depression

Having a chronic disease like type 2 diabetes is stressful. It can make you feel tired, angry, scared, resentful, or just plain sad.

Try not to worry; these feelings are normal. Being aware of and accepting these emotions may help you manage them better. The following sections address some of the emotions you may feel as you navigate life with diabetes.

Acknowledging diabetes burnout and stress

Diabetes distress, also called *diabetes burnout*, is a term used to describe those feeling of worry, fear, and frustration that come with managing a chronic disease like diabetes. It is quite common, with 18–45 percent of people with diabetes reporting diabetes distress.

You may feel frustrated with your new self-care routine, which can include being more conscientious about what you eat, exercising regularly, taking new medications, or checking your blood glucose. You may feel fearful about potential complications such as blindness or heart disease. You may worry about how you'll afford healthy foods, medications, or healthcare. You may feel like other people treat you unfairly because of your diabetes.

Stress is another common emotion for people with diabetes, and it can have similar triggers as those of diabetes burnout. Stress can affect your body and mind in various ways. For example, stress can raise your blood glucose or make it more challenging to stick to healthy foods or an exercise routine. Stress also interferes with sleep. You find out more about techniques for managing stress in Chapter 14.

TIP

Go easy on yourself. Recognize that other people with diabetes feel similarly. If you feel continually burned out or stressed, talk to your doctor or diabetes educator about your feelings. You may want to ask for a referral to a specialist such as a counselor or psychologist.

Recognizing depression

Depression is more common in people with diabetes. Although it may have similar symptoms to diabetes burnout and stress (see the preceding section), it is a distinct clinical diagnosis. If you feel sad or hopeless for more than 2 weeks, you may be suffering from depression.

Depression may or may not be related to diabetes. All kinds of things can cause depression, such as your life circumstances, the death of a person close to you, or medications you take for other conditions.

TIP

Talk to your doctor if you feel depressed. The doctor may prescribe an antidepressant or recommend that you see a psychiatrist, psychologist, social worker, or counselor. Depression is common and treatable, so don't be afraid to talk to your healthcare provider.

Being mindful of your emotions

Whatever you do, don't ignore your negative feelings about diabetes. Keep the following points in mind and talk to your doctor or a diabetes educator if you feel overwhelmed:

>> Diabetes distress is common and can make you feel angry, frustrated, fearful, or burned out.

>> Stress is common and can affect not just your feelings, but also your blood glucose and motivation to eat well and exercise regularly.

>> Depression is more common in people with diabetes.

>> Depression is a treatable condition with medications and/or therapy.

Talk to your doctor or nurse if you feel diabetes distress, stress, or signs of depression.

REMEMBER

Tuning In to Your Sexual Health

Feeling sexy and having sex are the spice of life, and they involve both your body and mind.

When it comes to your body, you want to keep your blood glucose on target to maintain healthy blood vessels. Blood vessel damage can affect a man's ability to have an erection. Blood vessel and nerve damage can hamper a woman's ability to reach orgasm or lead to vaginal dryness.

Keeping blood glucose low also helps prevent infections (flip back to the "Feeling Good in Your Skin" section for more about infections). Urinary tract or vaginal infections, which are more common in women with diabetes, can put a damper on sex.

As for your mind, remember that desire is a delicate balance between mind and body. How you feel about sex can be tied to your level of diabetes burnout, stress, depression — or anything else (see the "Coping with Burnout, Stress, and Depression" section earlier in this chapter for details about emotional health).

Talk to your healthcare provider if you're concerned about erectile dysfunction, orgasms, vaginal dryness, urinary or vaginal infections, or sexual desire. You may feel awkward at first. But don't be shy about expressing your feelings or concerns so you and your doctor can find the right treatments.

TIP

To keep your sexual embers burning, follow this advice:

>> Keep your blood glucose on target.

>> Lower your blood pressure and cholesterol, exercise, and eat nutritious foods.

>> Tell your doctor if you suspect a vaginal or urinary tract infection so you can get treatment.

>> Discuss erectile dysfunction with your healthcare provider.

>> Talk to your doctor about lack of desire or difficulty having orgasm.

Chapter 9

Women and Type 2 Diabetes

Women with diabetes can (and should) live vibrant, active lives. Nothing should stop women — especially diabetes. After all, you want to experience everything life serves up, whether you're diagnosed with diabetes when you're 30 or 70 or somewhere in between.

In this chapter, we walk you through the amazing female biological stages of your life as a woman with diabetes. And we also point out a few things to look out for along the way, like heart disease.

As you navigate the ups and downs of womanhood, the basic advice for managing type 2 diabetes applies: Eat healthy foods, exercise, lose weight if necessary, and take your recommended prescriptions. Your lifestyle and your medications will help you manage your blood glucose and feel great.

Read on to find out more about the unique experiences that make us women: menstruation, pregnancy, and menopause.

Being Mindful of Menstrual Cycles

No two women have the same menstrual cycle. Some women get their periods like clockwork every 28 days, while other women occasionally skip months. Some women have their periods for the average 7 days, while others may have bleeding for 3 days or 10 days. It all depends on your body — and your life at that moment.

Just as menstrual cycles differ, so do women's experiences with their diabetes during menstruation. It's totally unique. However, there are common themes for women with diabetes.

Watching for erratic numbers

Right before their periods, women with diabetes may notice their blood glucose numbers are erratic. The odd part: They could be high or low. Whatever the number, it's unexpected. And it may bum you out because it comes out of nowhere.

Why is your blood glucose wacky around this time? It may have something to do with fluctuations in the hormones progesterone and estrogen, as well as other factors such as premenstrual syndrome or symptoms, before you get your period.

Not every woman notices changes in her blood glucose during menstruation. So don't worry if you don't notice unexpected numbers. Just keep doing all the great things you're doing to manage your blood glucose.

The following section explains what to do if you experience unexpected highs or lows during your menstrual cycle.

Taking back control

If you consistently notice erratic blood glucose numbers right before your period begins, you may want to chart your blood glucose in relation to your menstrual cycle.

Make a spreadsheet or add an extra page in your logbook where you include the number of days in your menstrual cycle. Day 1 is the start of your period, and the last day is the final day before your next period. Write down or enter your blood glucose number(s) for each day in your cycle. Do it again the next month and the next month. After you have 3 or 4 months of data, take a look at your numbers and the days (Day 1, Day 13, Day 20) in your cycle. You may start to notice changes in your blood glucose just before your period.

TIP

If you experience highs, try to eat meals at your regularly planned times of the day and try not to skip meals. Maintaining a regular eating schedule can reduce big fluctuations in blood glucose and the accompanying mood swings. If you experience lows, try to eat more small meals throughout the day or eat an extra snack before you exercise.

Premenstrual syndrome (PMS; the physical and emotional symptoms that occur 1–2 weeks before a woman's period begins) is no fun. Just like anyone who experiences PMS, women with diabetes can take certain actions to feel better. Not every tactic works for everyone, but they're good tools to have at your disposal when the time comes.

TIP

If you experience PMS, try to limit sodium, which can cause bloating, by avoiding salty foods and reducing the number of meals you eat out. Use spices such as garlic powder, pepper, and cumin to give your foods a kick without salt. Take an extra walk at lunch or the stairs in the morning because exercise can improve both blood glucose and mood.

Talk to your healthcare provider about these changes and any concerns you have regarding your period and diabetes. She may have tips for you to manage highs and lows during your cycle.

TIP

Take time to discuss contraception with your provider. Women with diabetes have the same options for birth control as women without diabetes. Birth control pills, intrauterine devices (IUDs), implants, and barrier methods (diaphragms, condoms, spermicide) are all options. What you choose will depend on the needs of you and your partner. You'll also want to consider your medical history when choosing contraception. There are some risks and side effects associated with some forms of contraception, but the risk of an unplanned pregnancy generally outweighs the risk of any individual contraception.

Healthy Mom, Healthy Baby

Women with type 2 diabetes can have healthy pregnancies and babies. The goal is to keep blood glucose in your target range. We detail those specifics later in this section.

Keeping your blood glucose on target is particularly important when you're pregnant. You want to prevent complications for yourself and your baby. High blood glucose during pregnancy can put your baby at risk for becoming extremely large (called *macrosomia*) or having difficulty breathing or low blood glucose. It can also increase your baby's risk for developing type 2 diabetes during adolescence or adulthood.

REMEMBER

Gestational diabetes is different from type 1 and type 2 diabetes. It comes on during pregnancy and usually subsides after birth. However, women with gestational diabetes have a higher risk for type 2 diabetes in their lifetime.

Planning for pregnancy

If you have diabetes and you want to become pregnant, be sure to talk to your doctor and plan for this change. You want to be prepared and educated beforehand. Keeping your blood glucose in control before you become pregnant will help you have a healthy pregnancy and birth.

If you're thinking about becoming pregnant, talk to your healthcare provider so you can make a plan together. You may want to continue using birth control until your blood glucose is in a certain range. The American Diabetes Association recommends an A1C of less than 6.5 percent if possible before becoming pregnant.

TIP

Lose weight, exercise, and try to get your body in the best shape possible before you get pregnant. Quit smoking. Make sure you've had all your regular annual tests, including a dilated eye exam (because your eye health should be tracked closely during pregnancy).

TECHNICAL STUFF

Polycystic ovary syndrome (PCOS) is a hormone disorder that can cause abnormal menstrual cycles and infertility. PCOS patients also tend to be obese. Lifestyle changes and medications can help treat PCOS. Talk to your doctor if you suspect you may have it.

Taking care of yourself and your baby during pregnancy

During pregnancy, you may have to work harder than ever before to manage your blood glucose. Your blood glucose targets will probably be lower than they were before you became pregnant. This is to protect you and your baby from health risks during pregnancy.

For a woman, diabetes increases her risk for preeclampsia, which can raise blood pressure, cause dangerous swelling and weight gain, and can even be deadly. Pregnancy — with all its changing hormones — can also cause fluctuations in blood glucose. Blood glucose levels can be high or low, depending on the woman and the stage of her pregnancy. Insulin or other medication needs may change throughout this period and must be carefully monitored. Eye and kidney problems can get worse during pregnancy, so you and your healthcare team will want to monitor your health closely.

For a baby, high blood glucose and ketones can be passed from a pregnant woman to the developing fetus, and this can increase the risk for birth defects. The first trimester is a particularly important time because this is when the baby's organs are forming. High blood glucose in the first trimester increases the risk for birth defects and miscarriage. Babies can also be born particularly large (making delivery more dangerous for the baby and mother) and can have difficulty breathing.

Keeping your blood glucose in control during pregnancy reduces these risks for your baby. This is why it's so important to plan ahead for pregnancy — and have your A1C on target before you decide to conceive. Talk to your diabetes care provider about how to safely and thoughtfully plan for pregnancy.

The American Diabetes Association recommends an A1C of 6–6.5 percent during pregnancy. Your before-breakfast reading should be less than 96 mg/dL. You should strive for a reading of less than 141 mg/dL 1 hour after meals and less than 121 mg/dL 2 hours after meals. These are general recommendations, so please talk with your doctor about your individual goals.

Eating nourishing, wholesome foods is essential when you're pregnant. You're feeding your growing, hungry body and your growing, hungry baby. Select fresh fruits and vegetables, whole grains, and lean proteins (see Chapter 11 for more about nutritious eating when you have diabetes). There is never a more critical time to be mindful about what you put into your body.

TIP

The American Diabetes Association recommends that, during pregnancy, women with type 2 diabetes who are overweight gain 15–25 pounds and who are obese gain 10–20 pounds.

Exercise is just as important during pregnancy as it is before you become pregnant (see Chapter 13 for details on exercising when you have diabetes). The types of exercise you enjoy may change during pregnancy, especially during your final trimester. Some women prefer walking, swimming, and yoga. Ask your healthcare provider if you have questions about the type or intensity of exercise.

REMEMBER

Focus on your eyes. Women with diabetes are at risk for developing eye disease — or having it progress rapidly. You should have a dilated eye exam before you become pregnant or in the first trimester. Then you should have your eyes checked each trimester and for a year after you give birth.

WARNING

Not all medications are safe during pregnancy. Insulin is the preferred medication for managing blood glucose during pregnancy because it is safe and effective. You may need to switch to insulin if you take oral diabetes medications because they may not be approved for use during pregnancy. Many diabetes drugs have not been studied well, or at all, for use during pregnancy. If you already take insulin, you may need to change your dose or timing. Your doctor will advise you on this.

Tell your doctor about any other medications you're using, especially blood pressure and cholesterol drugs, because some are not recommended during pregnancy.

TIP

Try to breastfeed your baby if you can. It will benefit you and your newborn. Breast milk has amazing nutrients and antibodies. Breastfeeding also lowers your baby's risk for obesity later in life.

Screening for gestational diabetes

Gestational diabetes is high blood glucose that develops during pregnancy. It is separate from type 1 and type 2 diabetes, because it usually goes away after giving birth. But keep in mind that women with gestational diabetes are more likely to develop type 2 diabetes during their lifetimes.

You cannot get gestational diabetes *on top* of your type 2 diabetes. Instead, gestational diabetes is a diagnosis of high blood glucose during the second or third trimester of pregnancy. In some women, preexisting type 1 or type 2 diabetes will be diagnosed during their pregnancies; the presence of diabetes in the first trimester is thought to indicate preexisting diabetes, not gestational diabetes. This can be confusing because it might seem like gestational diabetes. However, these women will continue to manage and treat their diabetes after pregnancy.

All pregnant women are screened for gestational diabetes at 24–28 weeks using simple tests in which you drink a sugary liquid and a blood sample is tested afterward. Also, you may be tested at your initial prenatal visit if you have risk factors for type 2 diabetes.

In one test, you don't eat or drink anything with calories 8–14 hours before drinking the liquid. A provider takes a blood sample before, and then 1 and 2 hours after the drink. A fasting reading greater than 92 mg/dL, a 1-hour reading greater than 180 mg/dL or a 2-hour reading greater than 153 mg/dL could mean you have gestational diabetes.

In another test, you don't need to prepare at all before drinking the liquid. A provider takes a sample 1 hour after the drink. A high reading means you need to come back for a 3-hour test to diagnose gestational diabetes.

Women with gestational diabetes have the same blood glucose targets as women with type 1 or type 2 diabetes. Similar to women with type 2 diabetes, women with gestational diabetes have an increased risk of unusually large babies and the resulting complications during birth.

Women with gestational diabetes may need to change their meals or physical activity, or take insulin to manage their blood glucose during pregnancy. You'll work closely with your provider to come up with a plan for your pregnancy.

Delivering the baby

Women with type 2 diabetes or gestational diabetes are at risk for having larger babies and, therefore, more trauma during birth. However, keeping your blood glucose tightly managed during pregnancy can reduce this risk. Many women with diabetes deliver normal-weight babies.

As your delivery date nears, you'll work closely with your healthcare team to determine the best date and method for having your baby. They may analyze your blood glucose control, blood pressure, kidneys, and other health concerns. They'll also check your baby's health and size.

During delivery, the nurses and doctors will work to keep your blood glucose under control using insulin. You may not need as much insulin as you start active labor.

If your blood glucose was uncontrolled during pregnancy, your newborn baby could be at risk for low blood glucose (*hypoglycemia*). Your newborn will be tested after birth and then monitored in the hospital. The best way to prevent this is to manage your blood glucose closely during your pregnancy. After a baby has regular feedings, her blood glucose should return to normal levels, but it should be closely monitored. There is an increased risk for birth defects in babies born to women with preexisting diabetes that is not well controlled during pregnancy.

Postpartum

After giving birth, women with type 2 diabetes may have swings in their blood glucose. This could be confusing and unsettling, but it's normal as your body recovers from the amazing work of pregnancy and birth.

Talk to your provider about how to manage your blood glucose after pregnancy. You may need to test your blood glucose more often. It can be hard to focus on your own care when you have a new wee one, but make sure you're diligent about your own health. Just like any new mom, try to get as much sleep as possible and eat healthy meals. Check your blood glucose often to avoid episodes of low blood glucose.

Your provider will work with you to determine which diabetes medication to take after delivery. If you're breastfeeding, you'll want to consider that, too. Most diabetes medications are safe to take while breastfeeding, but review all your medication's safety profiles before you start breastfeeding your baby.

After giving birth, women with gestational diabetes may have normal blood glucose (and no longer need any medications). But they have a higher risk of gestational diabetes in subsequent pregnancies and a lifelong risk of developing type 2 diabetes. Therefore, women with gestational diabetes should have their blood glucose tested 1–3 months after giving birth, and then again every 1–3 years.

Breastfeeding

If you can, try to breastfeed your baby. The American Diabetes Association recommends that all women, whether they have type 1, type 2, or gestational diabetes, be encouraged to breastfeed. Breast milk provides essential nutrients and substances to boost your baby's immune system.

Breastfeeding can affect blood glucose in women with diabetes, so make sure that you talk to a dietitian or other healthcare provider about it. For example, you may need to eat a snack before or during breastfeeding to prevent a low. Breastfeeding can help women lose weight gained during pregnancy (a great thing), but you'll also want to make sure that you eat enough healthy foods and drinks to give you energy, keep you hydrated, and provide those essential vitamins and nutrients.

TIP

Every mom wants to lose the weight she gained during pregnancy. But it can be hard. Talk to a dietitian or other member of your team about your goals for losing weight after giving birth. You may need a new meal plan or exercise program that takes your goals and changed lifestyle into account.

Menopause Can Throw You for a Loop

Irregular periods, night sweats, and mood swings. Yes, these can be signs you're going through menopause. Another sign: unusual blood glucose numbers. Hormones can affect your blood glucose during menopause just as much as they do during your menstrual cycle.

Menopause is a natural part of life in which a woman's body makes less estrogen and progesterone, hormones that play key roles in menstruation. It marks the end of your body's ability to reproduce.

Menopause can last 8–10 years, although it varies for everyone. It's a process, not an event, and usually there are three stages: *perimenopause* (the time around the onset of menopause), menopause, and *postmenopause* (the time after menopause ends).

Many women begin menopause in their 40s, while others start in their 50s or 60s. The average age that an American woman has her last period is 51.

In the following sections, we cover the most common symptoms of menopause and how to deal with them when you have diabetes.

TIP

If you're considering hormone replacement therapy (HRT) to alleviate symptoms of menopause, talk to your doctor. HRT is a personal and nuanced issue.

Preparing for unusual numbers

Many women with diabetes have unexpected fluctuations in blood glucose as they go through menopause. Why? Hormones.

As you make less estrogen, your body may become less sensitive to insulin, and your blood glucose may be higher than usual. Even though you're doing the same things in terms of food, exercise, and medications, your blood glucose numbers can go up.

Another thing to consider is that you're not on your typical menstrual cycle. Perhaps you've always had regular periods and, therefore, a regular pattern of hormone changes throughout your cycle.

Menopause can be totally different. You may have longer periods or heavier bleeding. You may get your period all of a sudden after no bleeding for more than a year. Your body's hormones are changing, which affects your blood glucose, and there may be less predictability about how your body responds or how you feel.

TIP

To take action, check your blood glucose to see your actual numbers. Make sure you take your medications as prescribed, and ask your doctor if you feel like things aren't working. Take the time to take care of yourself by eating wholesome foods and exercising regularly.

Recognizing that mood swings are normal

Fluctuations in hormones and blood glucose (see the preceding section) don't happen in a vacuum. They happen in your body and mind. No wonder women going through menopause often experience mood swings and irritability. It's totally natural.

Your emotional state is intimately connected to changes in your body. It's directly related to hormones' effects on the brain.

The feeling of *going through* change can also mess with your emotions. Some people don't like the feeling of unpredictability that may occur during menopause. But remember that menopause is a transition that almost all women experience. Other women just like you are trying to manage their diabetes during this time.

TIP

Talk to a therapist or your healthcare provider if you feel like you need help. Seek out online or neighborhood support communities to find other women with diabetes going through menopause. (Chapter 15 offers more tips on finding support.) DiabetesSisters (www.diabetessisters.org) is an organization that offers articles and online education about women's health and diabetes.

Facing hot flashes and night sweats

Menopause is the main culprit of hot flashes and night sweats. They can both feel like moments of intense heat and sweating, followed by wetness and chills. Doctors believe that these unpleasant experiences occur because of fluctuating or decreasing estrogen levels, not because someone cranked up your house's thermostat. The change in estrogen may affect the part of the brain that regulates your body temperature, leading to feeling overheated.

Hot flashes can happen any time of day, while night sweats happen while you're sleeping. Although they're usually over after a few seconds or minutes, the after-effects such as sweaty clothes can be annoying.

Night sweats can be so intense that they wake you up from sleep, or you may wake up later with your pajamas drenched.

REMEMBER

The thing for women with diabetes to keep in mind is that hot flashes and night sweats can feel like low blood glucose. Why does that matter? Well, you wouldn't want to ignore a low by thinking it's just a hot flash. Therefore, you should always check your blood glucose just to be sure.

TIP

Try to wear breathable fabrics and dress in layers so you can take off clothes if you have a hot flash.

Coping with yeast infections

Yeast infections are more common in women going through menopause. As estrogen levels fall, the lining inside your vagina changes, making it more susceptible to infection. Symptoms include vaginal discharge, severe itching, and pain while urinating and during intercourse.

The fungus *Candida albicans* (the culprit behind yeast infections) likes to grow in warm, moist places and thrives when blood glucose levels are high. Women with diabetes going through menopause may find that they have more yeast infections.

TIP

To avoid yeast infections, wear clothes made of breathable fabrics to encourage airflow, and keep your genitals clean and dry. Try to avoid spermicide in condoms and personal sprays or douches.

Lots of women get yeast infections, so don't be shy about treating them. Over-the-counter antifungal creams may help in the early days of an infection, but if symptoms don't improve in a few days, call your doctor so she can write you a prescription.

Addressing sexual discomfort

Women going through menopause may find that sex is less comfortable than usual. Falling hormone levels change the walls of the vagina, and they may become thinner, drier, and irritated.

Added to this, high blood glucose could damage both nerves and blood vessels flowing to the vagina. Nerve damage could affect sensation in the vagina, impacting arousal or pleasure. Blood vessel damage could lessen blood flowing to the vagina and, therefore, arousal. To prevent these issues, try to keep your blood glucose and blood pressure in your target range by taking medications, eating healthy foods, and exercising regularly.

TIP

Use a lubricant like K-Y Jelly to make sex more enjoyable, or ask your doctor about estrogen creams that can treat vaginal dryness and itching.

What Every Woman with Diabetes Should Know

You know that your body, mind, and heart are unique and powerful. Maybe you read other parts of this chapter and thought, "That's never happened to me." Or maybe you thought, "Yeah, that's so true. Some of those things like mood swings and erratic blood glucose just happened last week." How your body reacts to menstruation, pregnancy, and menopause is totally dependent on you, your age, and the experiences you're going through in your life right now.

We can all agree that being a woman with diabetes has its challenges, but it also has its opportunities. Women with diabetes have never had so many options to practice safe sex and plan for pregnancy. More women than ever with diabetes are having babies. And women with diabetes going through menopause are finding other women like themselves to connect with online or in their communities.

As we wrap up this chapter, here's one more thing to keep in mind as a woman with diabetes.

Focus on your heart

You need to pay particular attention to your heart as a woman with diabetes. Let us say that again: Take care of your heart.

We used to think that women and men had the same risk of heart disease, but it's not true. Heart disease is the leading killer of women with diabetes. Women with diabetes have a 40 percent higher risk of heart disease than men with diabetes. Women with diabetes also have higher risk of stroke than men with diabetes.

In Chapter 8, we explain the importance of keeping your blood vessels healthy to prevent heart disease and stroke. You can keep your blood vessels healthy by losing weight and exercising. Eat nutritious foods that are low in sodium, saturated fat, and sugar (find out more about nutrition in Chapter 11). Take your medications as prescribed, including those for blood glucose, cholesterol, and blood pressure. Quit smoking.

Make sure you feel comfortable talking with your doctor about heart health. She should be just as focused as you are on preventing heart disease and stroke.

Know the signs

The most common sign of heart attacks in women are chest pressure or pain, the same as they are in men. However, other common symptoms of a heart attack such as shortness of breath, nausea, lightheadedness, discomfort in the lower chest or upper abdomen, and back or jaw pain seem to be more common in women. Extreme fatigue is also common.

Why do these other symptoms matter? It may be easier for women to dismiss these sometimes subtle and confusing symptoms as illness or an upset stomach.

Be aware of the signs of a heart attack. Don't dismiss symptoms that may not be as dramatic as clutching your chest and falling to the floor.

Call 911 immediately if you suspect a heart attack. There are effective treatments for heart attacks when caught early, and most people go on to lead healthy, productive lives.

Chapter **10**

Men and Type 2 Diabetes

Men with diabetes can live dynamic, productive, and healthy lives. If you're a man with diabetes, you may want to think about specific issues such as erectile dysfunction and low testosterone. In this chapter, we explore these male-specific concerns and offer suggestions about what you can do about them.

Not every man (or woman) is 100 percent comfortable talking about his health, particularly his sexual health. It's a taboo topic for some men who consider anything less than perfection a vulnerability or weakness.

However, being thoughtful and proactive about your health are some of the best things you can do for your body and mind. When you're proactive, you have the opportunity to build a healthcare team that you trust and can rely on for treatments and education. And of course, you should eat healthy foods, exercise, lose or maintain weight, and take medications to better manage your diabetes.

Some of the topics in this chapter may not be easy to discuss or contemplate because they relate to sex. However, keep in mind that you're not alone. Many men struggle with sexual issues, and the best way to find solutions is to be honest and forthcoming with your healthcare providers. Sex can be a healthy part of anyone's life, and complications from your diabetes shouldn't hold you back.

Addressing Erectile Dysfunction

Erectile dysfunction (ED), the inability to get or maintain an erection during sex (also called *impotence*), can be an uncomfortable topic to bring up because it's such a personal issue.

However, ED is definitely an issue for men with diabetes. For example, in a 2017 study in *Diabetic Medicine,* an analysis of previous studies found that erectile dysfunction affected more than half of men with diabetes. And men with diabetes were three and a half times more likely to experience erectile dysfunction than men without diabetes.

REMEMBER

ED varies in severity by individual. You may not experience complete ED each time you try to have an erection, but if you consistently have trouble getting or keeping an erection, talk to your physician.

The following sections explain the causes of and treatments for ED and give you some encouragement when you're ready to talk to your doctor and significant other about the condition.

Considering the causes

ED has more than one cause, which may include physical issues, psychological issues, or both. In other words, your mind *and* body could affect your ability to have an erection:

>> **Diabetes:** Men with type 2 diabetes have a greater risk of nerve damage and blood vessel damage. Both of these things can impact erections.

- *Nerve damage:* Also called *neuropathy,* nerve damage can cause ED because it may harm nerves that send signals to the penis. Keeping your blood glucose in your target range helps your nerves stay healthy over time.

- *Blood vessel damage:* Blood vessel damage can lessen blood flow to the penis and cause ED. Keeping your blood glucose on target, as well as quitting or not starting smoking, exercising, and losing weight can also improve your blood vessels and blood flow.

>> **Medications, alcohol, and other drugs:** Some medications — such as antidepressants, antihistamines, blood pressure medicines, and others — can also increase your risk for ED. Ask your doctor about these medications if you're concerned about ED. Recreational drugs such as alcohol can impact your erections, too.

>> **Low testosterone:** Low testosterone, which is discussed later in this chapter, can also contribute to ED.

>> **Your feelings about sex:** How you feel about sex can also impact your erections. Stress, anxiety, guilt, depression, or fear about *not* having an erection can affect your mood and function. Your relationship with your partner and what's going on with your life together can also affect erections. Don't discount your feelings about sex or what you think about during sex. These thoughts and feelings may make it harder to get and maintain an erection.

>> **Your age:** Your age can also affect how easily you get and maintain an erection. As all men age, not just men with diabetes, their risk of experiencing ED increases.

Treating erectile dysfunction

The good news is that treatments for ED abound. Prescription medications such as Viagra, Cialis, and Levitra can improve blood flow to your penis. The medications can be prescribed on a daily or an as-needed basis. Cialis for once daily use, for example, may be taken daily independent of the timing of sexual activity, whereas Viagra should be taken as needed before sexual activity. These treatments can be safe and effective for many men.

WARNING

However, when ED drugs and certain medications (particularly nitrates prescribed for chest pain) are taken together, the results can be fatal. Make sure your doctor and pharmacist know about all the medications you take.

A vacuum tube or pump can also draw blood into the penis if these medications don't work or aren't a safe option for you. Surgery with a penis implant is another treatment option.

Don't be embarrassed: Talking to your doctor

Talking to your physician is the best way to identify and treat ED. You may find it embarrassing or hard to admit the problem to someone else, but put aside your shyness. Your physician is on your side. He is a trained professional, and he should be able to offer education about and treatment for ED.

First, start by telling him your symptoms and concerns. He may ask you to describe your erections: their frequency, duration, and firmness. Don't forget to talk about your emotional health including depression, anxiety or dissatisfaction, or stress with your partner. Also, mention any physical changes you've noticed in your body. Be sure to tell your doctor about the medications that you're taking so you can rule those out as contributors. Lastly, discuss treatment options so you can find something that fits your lifestyle with a minimum of side effects.

REMEMBER

If, on occasion, you don't get or keep an erection, this does not mean you have ED. Most men experience this from time to time — it's considered a normal part of life.

Tackling the Problem of Low Testosterone

Testosterone is an important hormone for men. It does many things in the body, including regulating sexual desire or libido. In general, testosterone slightly and gradually declines after middle age. Moderate alcohol consumption and regular opioid use may decrease testosterone levels.

Some men have low testosterone, which can contribute to low sexual desire, ED, depression, low energy, increases in body fat, and loss of muscle mass. Men with type 2 diabetes are twice as likely to have low testosterone as men without diabetes. Overweight men are also predisposed to lower testosterone.

Low testosterone shares many symptoms with other problems, but a simple blood test can diagnose it. If you're experiencing symptoms such as a lower libido, decreased energy and mood, or ED, tell your healthcare provider. A large deficiency in testosterone may cause your doctor to evaluate you for underlying conditions, such as problems with your pituitary gland or other organs, that may have gone unnoticed.

Hormone treatments such as gels, patches, and injections boost testosterone. If you want more details, ask for a referral to an endocrinologist or urologist who specializes in treating low testosterone.

Focusing on Emotional and Sexual Health

Your brain is an important sexual organ. It's tied to your libido, but also the nerves and blood vessels that flow to your penis and other areas of arousal.

Physical issues such as damage to your blood vessels or nerves can affect your enjoyment of and fulfillment during sex. These real physical changes can make you feel negative or less confident about sex in general. And these emotions can affect sexual desire.

TIP

Don't leave your partner in the dark in terms of your emotional or sexual health. It can be hard to bring up, but talking and intimacy are a foundation of healthy relationships.

Talking to a counselor or mental health professional may also help. Ask your physician or diabetes educator about these options.

Paying Attention to Heart Health

Heart and blood vessel health is important for men with type 2 diabetes. They have double the risk of heart attacks and other blood vessel diseases than men without diabetes.

ED and the hardening of arteries (a condition known as *atherosclerosis*) are related, so if you have ED, you may want to ask your physician about your risk for cardiovascular disease, too.

TIP

To reduce your risk of heart disease, lose weight or maintain a healthy weight, exercise, eat nutritious and wholesome foods, lower your blood pressure, keep your blood lipids on target, and try a smoking cessation program if you use tobacco.

There's a lot more information to know about heart health when you have diabetes. Check out Chapter 8 for details on the importance of keeping your blood vessels healthy to prevent heart disease and stroke.

4

Eating Healthy and Staying Active

Discover how carbs, protein, and fat fit into a balanced diet and how a dietitian can help you make healthy food choices.

Understand how choosing a variety of foods, eating the right portion sizes for you, and creating meal plans lead to better health and nutrition.

Start sitting less and moving more to jumpstart your fitness.

Chapter **11**

Brushing Up on Nutrition and Food Basics

You know it, and we know it: Eating healthy foods isn't always easy. We all struggle to make nutritious choices given the abundance of processed convenience foods in America.

Don't despair. When you know that healthy options are available, you'll find foods that you love to eat. Think of having diabetes as an opportunity to embrace healthy foods and choices. It's a cornerstone of your diabetes care.

In this chapter, we explain why working with a dietitian can be beneficial when you're changing your eating habits. Then we give you the background on the three basic nutrients: carbohydrates, protein, and fat. Each group has some superstar foods that you should make sure to include in your diet.

This chapter also goes deep into food labels and how to use them to make healthy choices. Along the way, you find out about three S's to cut back on: sugar, soda, and sodium. We wrap things up by talking about refreshing drinks to enjoy with meals or on their own.

Knowing the Difference a Dietitian Can Make

Your number-one resource for healthy eating is your dietitian. Everyone with diabetes should have access to a dietitian to come up with a personalized meal plan. Notice we didn't say *diet*; we said *meal plan*. There's no one-size-fits-all diet for people with diabetes. (Find out more about meal plans and why diets aren't prescribed for people with diabetes in Chapter 12.)

You may not have met with a dietitian before you were diagnosed with diabetes. You may think you don't need one, especially if you don't have to follow a certain diet. But dietitians are an excellent resource to help you determine a meal plan that's right for *you.*

So, what is a dietitian? An expert in food and nutrition. A *dietitian* is a professional trained in providing medical nutrition therapy. In other words, a dietitian can help you learn about nutrition, set healthy eating goals, or lose weight to help manage chronic diseases like diabetes.

The term *dietitian* is a broad umbrella, and dietitians help all kinds of people, including those who have cancer or eating disorders or heart disease. You may want to find a dietitian who specializes in helping people with diabetes.

What to look for in a dietitian

Dietitians study and earn credentials just like other health professionals. When you're looking for a dietitian, look for the letters RD or RDN.

A *registered dietitian* (RD) or *registered dietitian nutritionist* (RDN) is a health professional who helps people determine the best path forward for meal planning, nutrition, and weight management. RDs and RDNs are accredited by the Commission on Dietetic Registration.

Separately, most states have laws that regulate how dietitians practice in those states. For example, the state of Texas has an agency that oversees dietitians that is distinct from the state of Connecticut. You may see the letters LDN after a dietitian's name, which stands for *licensed dietitian nutritionist* or CDN, which stands for *certified dietitian nutritionist.*

Check out the website of the Academy of Nutrition and Dietetics (www.eatright. org) for more information about types of dietitians and how to find one in your area.

TIP

In addition to making sure your dietitian is a credentialed RD or RDN, you may also want to look for a registered dietitian who is a certified diabetes educator (CDE). A dietitian who is a CDE has additional training in diabetes management and can help you with your general diabetes care.

Ask your healthcare provider for a recommendation; he or she is probably your best resource for finding an experienced and available professional in your area. Local hospitals should also have resources for finding dietitians in your community.

What dietitians do

Dietitians are trained to educate and counsel people about food and nutrition to help people manage medical conditions like diabetes. They can also help you create a healthy meal plan that fits your goals, lifestyle, and culture.

For example, you may have a goal of losing weight. A dietitian can help you come up with a meal plan that cuts back on calories without leaving you hungry. Or you may want to reduce your sodium because your blood pressure is high. A dietitian can give you tips for choosing foods with less salt.

Some people with diabetes may cook for their whole family, so making separate meals may not be practical — or economical. Other people may work two jobs, so cooking dinner at home isn't always an option. Discuss these lifestyle considerations with your dietitian so together you can devise strategies that work for you.

And don't forget to talk about your culture and history with food. After all, your grandma's recipe for enchiladas may be integral to how you celebrate and cook for your family today. You can still eat food that has cultural or personal meaning, but you may need to substitute ingredients or enjoy these treats more selectively.

TIP

In addition to everything we've already mentioned, dietitians can help you:

>> Learn about the basics of nutrition and food

>> Create a personalized meal plan

>> Choose foods that you're passionate about and love to eat

>> Fit those foods into your meal plan in healthy ways

>> Make good choices at the grocery store

>> Make healthy decisions when you're eating out

>> Turn a less healthy recipe into a healthy recipe with flavor and punch

>> Discover new cookbooks, recipes online, or food apps for your phone

>> Understand how foods affect your blood glucose

Dietitians are there to listen so don't be afraid to ask questions about food and nutrition and how it relates to your goals. It's part of the learning process.

When to see a dietitian

You should have access to a dietitian when you're first diagnosed with diabetes — and then if you can, every year after that.

Your initial visit may be about an hour because the dietitian will evaluate your needs and you'll work together on a meal plan. Follow-up visits may only last 30 minutes.

Try not to look at your visit to a dietitian as a one-and-done experience. You should meet with a dietitian every year to talk about changes to your goals, health, lifestyle, and likes and dislikes. A dietitian can help you stay on track and sustain healthy goals. In the follow-up visits, you may not need a complete overhaul, but you can probably benefit from a meal plan tune-up (see Chapter 12 for details about meal plans).

Your first appointment with a dietitian should take place shortly after you're diagnosed with diabetes. However, you should call a dietitian when any of the following applies:

>> It's been a year since you last saw a dietitian.

>> Your meals bore you.

>> You dread cooking or shopping for healthy foods.

>> Your blood glucose or weight has become more difficult to control than usual.

>> You're changing your medications, including starting insulin.

>> You have other health concerns such as high blood pressure, cholesterol, or kidney disease.

>> You're pregnant or trying to become pregnant.

>> You're entering menopause.

People with diabetes may be referred for diabetes education (and specifically medical nutrition therapy) at four critical times: at diagnosis, on an annual basis, when factors complicate your ability to take care of yourself, and during transitions in care such as changes to your doctors or insurance.

Paying for dietitian visits

Many people don't know that seeing a dietitian may be covered under health insurance if you have diabetes. It falls under the category of "medical nutrition therapy."

TIP

Call your health insurance company to see if medical nutrition therapy for diabetes is covered under your plan. You will need a prescription for medical nutrition therapy from your healthcare provider, and try to see an RD, RDN, or CDE covered by your plan.

Medicare Part B covers medical nutrition therapy and related services for people with diabetes. This may include an initial nutrition and lifestyle assessment, one-on-one nutritional counseling, and follow-up visits. Sometimes Medicare will cover medical nutrition therapy through telehealth (real-time audio and video) if you live in a rural area.

If you have Medicare Part B, you'll also need a referral from your doctor for medical nutrition therapy. Check out www.medicare.gov for more information.

Many states also cover medical nutrition therapy under their Medicaid programs. Call your Medicaid program or ask your doctor to see if you qualify.

TIP

To increase the chances of having the cost of your dietitian visits covered by your health insurance, follow these tips:

>> Call your health insurance provider and ask whether your plan covers medical nutrition therapy for diabetes.

>> If you have coverage, ask about specifics you'll need to provide such as a referral from your doctor or other paperwork.

>> Ask whether your nutrition provider can submit directly to your health insurance or whether you'll need to submit a claim each time.

>> If you're denied, don't give up. Resubmit your claim and ask for a review, in writing. Follow up with phone calls and write down the names of people you talk with and the dates so you have them for your records.

Calories Count

Calories sometimes have a bad reputation. But step back and think about what a calorie *is*.

A *calorie* is a measurement of the amount of energy in a food. It's that simple.

If your goal is to maintain your weight, you will aim to eat the same amount of calories that you burn though exercise and daily activity. It's all about calories in balanced with calories out.

If your goal is to lose weight, you will aim to eat fewer calories and burn more calories through exercise and daily activity.

Some types of food such as fats have more calories per bite than other types of foods such as carbohydrates and proteins. Find out more about these nutrients in the following sections.

The American Diabetes Association does not recommend that people with diabetes eat a certain number of calories per day or necessarily count their calories. However, you and your dietitian may decide that it's important for you to count calories based on your weight, age, activity, goals, and health. If you're trying to lose weight, you may work with a dietitian to develop a meal plan that restricts your calories.

Regardless of whether you're counting calories, it's sometimes helpful to know whether you're eating something with a lot of calories (like a 1,000-calorie fast-food burger) or fewer calories (like 85 calories in a dozen steamed shrimp).

To know how many calories are in a food, check out the food label on the package (we give you the lowdown on food labels later in the chapter). If the item doesn't have a food label, as in the case of fresh fruits and vegetables, meat from the butcher, and many other foods, you're going to have to work harder to get that information. A great resource for calorie and nutrient information is the U.S. Department of Agriculture's (USDA) Food Composition Databases where you can search by food item or food group: https://ndb.nal.usda.gov/ndb. You can also look on Google Play or iTunes for apps that tell you the calories and nutrition information for foods.

Nutrients: Carbohydrates, Protein, and Fat

When you think about food groups, maybe you imagine a food pyramid from elementary school. The pyramid base was made up of a giant foundation of loaves of bread holding up smaller blocks of broccoli and carrots and other vegetables on one side and bananas, grapes, oranges, and other fruits on the other, with yet another smaller block with a glass of milk and slices of Swiss cheese above it.

Well, things have changed a bit since then. No one is going to make a meal plan out of a giant foundation of bread, as much as we may enjoy it. Today the USDA uses a program called MyPlate, which recommends eating a variety of nutritional foods in more balanced amounts. MyPlate is designed for the general population to follow.

You can think of food as fitting into three main groups of nutrients: carbohydrates, protein, and fat. These are called macronutrients, and you need them for your body to do all its important work.

Carbohydrates, protein, and fat are found in all different foods, not just one type. Some foods may have only one of these nutrients, while other foods may have all three.

Try to eat a variety of foods to help you get all these nutrients. Here's a quick breakdown of how different foods fit into the categories:

>> **Carbohydrates:** Vegetables; fruits; beans; whole-grain cereals, pastas, and breads; and milk and yogurt

>> **Proteins:** Meat such as beef, pork, poultry (chicken and turkey), fish, beans, lentils, and soy products

>> **Fats:** Oils, margarine, butter, and cream

In the following sections, we walk through carbohydrates, protein, and fat in detail. You find out more about which foods make up each category and which types and what portions of those foods to include.

Carbohydrates 101

Carbohydrates provide big-time energy for your body. Your body breaks down carbohydrates into glucose, which is then absorbed into your bloodstream. Your blood glucose will start to rise within 15 minutes of eating carbohydrates.

REMEMBER

Carbohydrates are the main trigger for blood glucose rising after eating. Therefore, think about carbohydrates when developing a meal plan, which you find out more about in Chapter 12.

The American Diabetes Association does not recommend any specific number of carbohydrates that people with type 2 diabetes should eat each day. Instead, eat carbohydrates in moderation just like other nutrients such as protein and fat.

TIP

Work with a dietitian to come up with a personalized strategy for choosing and managing carbohydrates. You can find out more about carb counting and low-carb eating in Chapter 12.

Types of carbohydrates

Many, many foods such as vegetables, fruits, bread, pasta, popcorn, and beans are made up of carbohydrates. These carbohydrates have essential fiber, vitamins, and minerals. They're often easily absorbed, making them great sources of energy.

Filling up on veggies

Nonstarchy vegetables are perhaps the most nutrient-rich, low-calorie carbohydrates. They're chock-full of vitamins, minerals, and fiber. They're low in calories, so you can eat more of them than other foods. In general, dietitians recommend three to five servings of nonstarchy vegetables a day.

Asparagus, radishes, cucumbers, carrots, broccoli, tomatoes, peppers, spinach, and red and green lettuce are all nonstarchy vegetables. There are dozens more, including these, which are not as common:

>> Whole artichokes or artichoke hearts

>> Beets

>> Brussels sprouts

>> Cauliflower

>> Jicama

>> Kale

Eating these vegetables fresh is a great option. Go to the produce section of your grocery store and see what's in season. Or better yet, go to your local farmers' market. You may be surprised at the variety and beauty of the selections.

Don't worry if you can't eat fresh vegetables all the time. Frozen and canned vegetables are great options, too. After all, no one can dispute the ease of heating up frozen broccoli on a weeknight. And frozen vegetables are just as nutritious as their fresh counterparts — good news if you live in a northern climate where growing seasons are shorter.

TIP

Canned or frozen vegetables can be more affordable than fresh ones. Try to avoid packaged vegetables with added sauces or salt. For example, some frozen vegetables have sauce packets and some canned vegetables have added salt. Sometimes manufacturers will add sodium to improve flavor. However, you can also look for canned and frozen vegetables without added salt. They may even explicitly say on the label "no salt added." Now, more than ever, low-sodium options are available in grocery aisles. We tell you more about reading food labels later in this chapter. Lowering your sodium intake can help lower your blood pressure and improve your heart health.

Starchy vegetables also provide benefits and include potatoes, corn, beans, and peas. They're a great source of vitamins and minerals. Less common starchy vegetables that are packed with vitamins include

>> Butternut squash

>> Parsnips

>> Plantains

>> Sweet potatoes and yams

You can substitute legumes and beans for a starchy vegetable. Some to try include

>> Black-eyed peas

>> Garbanzo beans

>> Kidney beans

>> Lentils

TIP

Eating three to five servings of vegetables a day is fantastic, but you can eat many more if they're nonstarchy vegetables like carrots, cucumbers, radishes, and tomatoes.

Adding grains to your meal

Carbohydrates are found in grains such as rice and wheat, and in all types of breads, pastas, and tortillas.

REMEMBER

Whole grains are a better choice than refined grains because they contain more fiber, vitamins, minerals, and other awesome nutrients. To get the full benefits, choose foods that list whole grains as a first ingredient.

TECHNICAL STUFF

What makes a whole grain whole? A whole grain contains the entire grain kernel, which includes the bran, germ, and endosperm.

Whole wheat is probably the most famous type of whole grain, but you can choose from oodles of other grains such as brown rice and quinoa. Just take a look at all your options:

>> Barley

>> Brown rice

>> Corn, including popcorn and whole cornmeal

>> Farro

>> Oats, including oatmeal

>> Quinoa

>> Wild rice

Enjoying fruit in limited amounts

Fruits are another yummy and nutritious carbohydrate packed with vitamins, minerals, and fiber. Fruits also contain a naturally occurring sugar called *fructose*.

You want to choose fruit in moderation as part of your meal plan.

Just like vegetables, choose fruits from the fresh produce section of your grocery store or farmers' market. Could there be anything simpler than biting into a crisp apple for a snack?

Frozen fruits are a handy, healthy addition to smoothies and other desserts or as a cereal topping. You can also thaw frozen fruits and eat them that way. Dried fruits (in small portions) are super snacks to have on hikes or in the car. Avoid fruits soaked in sugary syrups, such as some canned fruit or packaged fruit cups.

Keep two or three of these fruits on hand for when a case of the munchies hits. When one goes out of season, switch to one coming into season:

>> Blueberries

>> Apples

>> Pears

>> Peaches

>> Honeydew melon

>> Kiwi

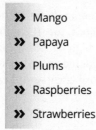

>> Mango

>> Papaya

>> Plums

>> Raspberries

>> Strawberries

The lowdown on sugar

Sugar is another carbohydrate. It's often held up as one of those foods that people with diabetes shouldn't eat. Or even worse, some people think sugar causes diabetes. These things simply aren't true.

Sugar is dangerous when people eat too much of it *and* they eat it instead of other nutritious foods. In other words, it's easy to fill up on sugar, and not have room for the good stuff. Many people do this by drinking large quantities of sugary soft drinks.

TECHNICAL STUFF

A growing body of scientific evidence says people should avoid drinking sugar-sweetened beverages so they don't gain weight and exacerbate other problems such as high blood pressure and cholesterol. The American Diabetes Association recommends avoiding sugar-sweetened drinks.

Think beyond the sugar in a bowl on your kitchen table. It's probably not your main source of sugar. Added sugar is the sneaky culprit.

WARNING

Added sugar is almost everywhere. It's in the desserts we enjoy like cookies, cake, and ice cream. It's in drinks like soda, sport drinks, energy drinks, and sweetened iced tea. It can even be in snacks like crackers, bread, and granola bars. We explain how to find added sugars in the "Nutrients up next" section later in this chapter.

Limit your amount of added sugar, and that includes in all those foods in the preceding paragraph. The American Heart Association recommends consuming no more than 100 calories (6 teaspoons) of added sugar for women and 150 calories (9 teaspoons) of added sugar for men each day.

Keep in mind an average 12-ounce can of soda (not the super-size from the local convenience store) has 8 teaspoons of added sugar.

Talk to your dietitian about how to make healthy choices about sugar. You can discuss how to include desserts in your meal plan by paying attention to your carbohydrates and calories.

High-fructose corn syrup is a type of sugar commonly found in sodas and other sweetened beverages, but it's in lots of other foods, too. It's quite similar to table sugar. There isn't a consensus about whether high-fructose corn syrup is worse than other sugars. However, it should be considered an added sugar just like any other. Too much sugar, including high-fructose corn syrup, can lead to health problems such as weight gain.

Artificial sweeteners

Artificial sweeteners, or nonnutritive sweeteners, are a way to sweeten foods and beverages with fewer calories than sugar. Artificial sweeteners are also called *low-calorie sweeteners* or *sugar substitutes.* They're sweeter than sugar, so you need less of them to get the same level of sweetness.

For some people with diabetes who are used to eating sugar-sweetened products, artificial or nonnutritive sweeteners may be an acceptable substitute for calorie-containing sweeteners (such as sugar, honey, and agave syrup) when consumed in moderation. Nonnutritive sweeteners do not appear to have a significant effect on blood glucose control, but according to the American Diabetes Association, they may help people with diabetes reduce their calorie and carbohydrate intake. You may have heard negative reports about artificial sweeteners suggesting that they cause cancer. Studies have not shown an association between artificial sweeteners and cancer in humans.

The U.S. Food and Drug Administration (FDA) is responsible for regulating artificial sweeteners because they're considered food additives. The FDA has approved six artificial sweeteners as food additives: acesulfame potassium, advantame, aspartame, neotame, saccharin, and sucralose.

Two other artificial sweeteners have the designation Generally Recognized as Safe (GRAS). They are luo han guo extract and stevia. Manufacturers can market these sweeteners without FDA approval.

You may not be familiar with the names of artificial sweeteners we've included here, but you've heard the brand names.

>> **Acesulfame potassium:** Sunett, Sweet One

>> **Aspartame:** Equal, Nutrasweet

>> **Neotame:** Neotame

>> **Saccharin:** Sweet'N Low, Sugar Twin

>> **Stevia:** PureVia, Stevia in the Raw, Sun Crystals, SweetLeaf, Truvia

>> **Sucralose:** Splenda

WARNING

Agave nectar is a sweetener that comes from the agave plant. It's often marketed for people with diabetes. However, agave nectar has the same effect on blood glucose as other sugars.

Proteins 101

Proteins are essential nutrients that help our bodies repair themselves and build new tissues and muscles. Proteins also transport oxygen to cells through our bloodstream. Normally, your body won't use protein for energy unless you don't have enough carbohydrates and fats available.

The American Diabetes Association does not recommend any specific amount of protein that people with type 2 diabetes should eat each day. Instead, eat protein in moderation just like other nutrients like carbohydrates and fat. Work with a dietitian to come up with a personalized strategy for incorporating healthy proteins into meals.

You can find protein in meat, fish and shellfish, eggs, milk, and other dairy foods. Vegetables, grains, and legumes also have protein. Nuts are a wonderful source of protein, too.

The key to choosing healthy protein foods is choosing ones low in saturated fats (find out more about fats in the following section). Select lean cuts of beef, pork, poultry, and seafood.

Fish, shellfish, and eggs are super sources of protein, and they also have omega-3 fats, which can reduce your risk for cardiovascular disease. You've probably tried salmon, but how about rainbow trout, sardines, or albacore tuna? Try to eat two to three servings of fish a week.

When you want a change from meat, fish, and eggs, prepare one of these shellfish, all of which are full of protein:

>> Clams

>> Crab

>> Oysters

>> Scallops

>> Shrimp

Milk and dairy foods like yogurt and cheese also have lots of protein — and calcium to boot. Milk also has carbohydrates, in addition to protein. Choose low-fat versions that have less saturated fat.

Nuts such as almonds and pistachios are protein power foods. They curb hunger while providing fiber and protein. And don't forget about seeds such as pine nuts and sunflower or pumpkin seeds. Nuts and seeds are also super for snacking. You can also sprinkle them on yogurt in the morning, dinner salads, or dessert sorbet.

Fats 101

Fat is the third essential nutrient we want to cover. Wait, fat is a nutrient? Those two words don't seem like they should go together. Actually, your body needs small amounts of fat to survive.

In fact, your body makes its own type of fat called *cholesterol.* Your body uses cholesterol to rebuild membranes that protect cells and to help your cells send signals to one another. Cholesterol is also used to make hormones.

Because your body makes its own fat (cholesterol), you only need to eat small amounts of fat. We'll say that again: You only need to eat a little fat.

WARNING

Many people eat way too much fat. Eating too much fat can clog your arteries and lead to heart disease and stroke.

The American Diabetes Association doesn't recommend a specific amount of fat that people with type 2 diabetes should eat each day. Instead, focus on eating healthy fats (see the next section).

Work with a dietitian to come up with a personalized strategy for incorporating healthy fats and reducing unhealthy fats in your meals.

Choosing healthy fats

Healthy fats are unsaturated fats, which include monounsaturated and polyunsaturated fats. Unsaturated fats are thought to be good for your heart and can reduce inflammation.

Nuts such as almonds, peanuts, walnuts, and pistachios are a good source of monounsaturated fat. Olives and sesame seeds have monounsaturated fats.

Don't forget avocados. Plant oils such as olive oil, canola oil, and peanut and other nut oils are good sources of polyunsaturated fats.

Check out the following list of foods that contain healthy fats. Some of them might surprise you.

>> Avocados

>> Flaxseed and flaxseed oil

>> Olives

>> Pumpkin seeds

>> Sesame seeds

>> Walnuts

Healthy fats also include omega-3 fats, which are an especially healthy type of fat. Fish and shellfish are the best sources of omega-3 fats, and fatty fish like salmon, tuna, and sardines are winners. Walnuts and flaxseeds provide omega-3 fats, too.

Studies have shown that consuming omega-3 fats reduces the risk of cardiovascular disease in people with and without diabetes. For this reason, the American Diabetes Association recommends that people with diabetes eat two or more 4-ounce servings of fatty fish a week. Try one of these:

>> Albacore tuna

>> Herring

>> Mackerel

>> Rainbow trout

>> Salmon

>> Sardines

The American Diabetes Association does not recommend omega-3 fats in the form of supplements for people with diabetes. Instead, try to eat these fats from fish, shellfish, walnuts, flaxseed, or other foods.

Avoiding unhealthy fats

Unhealthy fats are saturated fats and trans fats. Saturated and trans fats can raise your cholesterol, clog your blood vessels, and put you at greater risk for heart disease and stroke. Unhealthy fats harm blood vessels throughout your body, so, as a person with diabetes, be especially careful about eating too much.

TIP

Reading food labels is an integral skill for reducing unhealthy fats such as saturated and trans fat. We give you all sorts of important facts about food labels in the "Finding Nutrition Facts on Food Labels" section later in this chapter.

Steering clear of saturated fats

Saturated fats are found mostly in meat and dairy foods, such as butter, whole milk, yogurt, cheese, ice cream, and meats. But that doesn't mean you can't eat these foods. Instead, choose healthier versions. The following foods are full of saturated fat:

>> Chicken and turkey skin

>> Coconut oil

>> Heavy cream sauces

>> Palm oil

>> Sour cream

WARNING

You may notice that coconut oil is everywhere lately. It's sometimes dubbed as a "healthy alternative" because it has been shown to raise the good kind of cholesterol in the body. However, coconut is also full of unhealthy saturated fat. In fact, it has 82 percent saturated fat (compared to butter's 63 percent). It may be okay to use sometimes, but it's not recommended to start substituting coconut oil for other healthier alternatives like olive oil. Talk to your dietitian if you have questions about using coconut oil.

Select lean types of meat such as chicken or select cuts of meat that contain less fat. Before you prepare meat or as you're eating it, cut the fat off and discard it.

Tracking down trans fats

You'll find some trans fats in meat and dairy products, but mostly trans fats are manufactured in the laboratory and added to foods. Trans fats were originally added to keep packaged foods fresh on the shelf longer. However, we now know that eating trans fats isn't healthy and we should try to avoid them.

Manufacturers are now required to label foods that contain trans fats. You know a food contains trans fat when you see the ingredients "hydrogenated oil" or "partially hydrogenated oil" on the package. It's also listed in the nutrition facts.

Finding Nutrition Facts on Food Labels

Everyone knows foods have a nutrition label. But do you actually read it?

If you have diabetes, now's the time to start. Food labels are a good source of information about the foods you eat. They're packed with facts about calories, carbohydrates, protein, fats, and added sugars.

The FDA recently tweaked the design and updated the labels to highlight new science. Most food labels should reflect these changes in the coming years but, in the meantime, you may see both the old and the new versions. Here's the skinny on what to pay special attention to when you read a food label.

Paying attention to number of servings and serving size

Servings per container and serving size are the first things you should look at on the food label (see Figure 11-1). Together, they tell you how to read the rest of the food label. In the new food label design, both servings per container and serving size are in larger, bolder lettering than before.

Nutrition Facts

8 servings per container

Serving size	**2/3 cup (55g)**

Amount per serving

Calories	**230**

	% Daily Value*
Total Fat 8g	**10%**
Saturated Fat 1g	**5%**
Trans Fat 0g	
Cholesterol 0mg	**0%**
Sodium 160mg	**7%**
Total Carbohydrate 37g	**13%**
Dietary Fiber 4g	**14%**
Total Sugars 12g	
Includes 10g Added Sugars	**20%**
Protein 3g	
Vitamin D 2mcg	10%
Calcium 260mcg	20%
Iron 8mg	45%
Potassium 235mg	6%

*The % Daily Value (DV) tells you how much a nutrient in a serving of food contributes to a daily diet. 2,000 calories a day is used for general nutrition advice.

FIGURE 11-1: A food label contains all sorts of nutrition information.

Courtesy of the American Diabetes Association

First, look at the servings per container. Does it say 1 or 3? Many packages have more than one serving. However, it's easy to ignore the fine print because eating the whole package seems like the right size. Beware, especially when you're hungry.

Servings per container tells you how many servings are in the entire package. For example, you'll want to know whether the bag of popcorn you bought contains one serving or more than one serving. You may plan to eat the whole bag for a snack, but it may actually have three servings of popcorn.

Next, look at the serving size. If it's ½ cup, then all of the nutrients and calories listed on the label pertain to that serving.

Usually, the information listed on the food label refers to one serving. Some labels may have information for the whole package in a side-by-side format.

If you eat more than one serving from the whole bag of popcorn, you'll need to multiply the nutrition ingredients, including calories, by the number of servings you eat.

Keeping track of calories

The second thing to look at on a food label is the Calories line. You may first notice that the word *calories* is enlarged. The number of calories per serving is enlarged too (refer to Figure 11-1).

Food labels have been redesigned to show the importance of calories when thinking about food. In general, 100 calories per serving is a moderate amount and 400 calories per serving is high, according to the FDA. Think about your personal total calorie goals for the day to put these numbers in perspective.

Remember that the calories *per serving* are listed. So, if you have three servings in a popcorn bag and you eat the whole bag, you'll need to multiply the calories by 3 to figure out how many calories you consumed.

Nutrients up next

The middle section of the food label lists information about nutrients: carbohydrates, fat, and protein (refer to Figure 11-1). (Check out the earlier sections in this chapter on these nutrients.)

The food label lists the amount of nutrients per serving, as both a weight and a percent daily value.

Weights are measured in grams and may not mean much to you. (Just how much is 30 grams of fat anyway?)

What is percent daily value? *Percent daily value* tells you how much of a nutrient in a serving contributes to your daily diet. It's a guideline that tells you, for example, you're eating a ton of fat or just a little fat. The percent daily value will probably mean more to you than the nutrient's weight per serving. If you see that one serving of a food contains 20 percent of the recommended daily amount of fat (that's one-fifth of the day's total), you might rethink your choice of snack.

In general, 5 percent of a nutrient is low and 20 percent of a nutrient is high per serving, according to the FDA.

Fats are listed first: total fat, saturated fat, and trans fat. *Remember:* Try to avoid saturated fat and trans fat because they can increase the risk of cardiovascular disease.

Cholesterol and sodium are next. Choose foods with low numbers to keep your blood vessels healthy. You'll find out more about reducing sodium later in the chapter.

As a person with diabetes, pay attention to the carbohydrates section. If you're following a meal plan in which you count or reduce carbohydrates, this section of the food label is a great resource. (Find out more on carbohydrate counting in Chapter 12.)

Pay special attention to a new line called "Added Sugars." *Added sugars* refer to the sugars or syrups that are added to a food during processing or preparation, not the sugars that naturally occur in certain foods. Eating too much added sugar isn't good for you because you fill up with sugar instead of eating more nutritious foods. Try to keep that number low by avoiding foods with added sugars.

Other important vitamins such as vitamin D, calcium, iron, and potassium are listed on food labels. Dietary fiber is on there, too. The FDA says most Americans do not get enough of these nutrients, and studies have shown that these nutrients can decrease the risk of high blood pressure, cardiovascular disease, osteoporosis, and anemia. Try to get 100 percent of the daily value of these vitamins and nutrients a day.

Table 11-1 gives you a quick rundown of nutrients to get more of and ones to avoid.

TABLE 11-1

Food Label Categories

Nutrients to Embrace	Nutrients to Avoid
Vitamin D	Saturated fat
Calcium	Trans fat
Iron	Sodium
Potassium	Added sugars
Dietary fiber	

Listing ingredients: Most to least

Ingredients are usually listed right below the nutrition facts panel, although this can vary. The ingredients section lists the main ingredient first and the rest of the ingredients in descending order by weight.

TIP

Look for wholesome, nutritious ingredients listed first. For example, whole-grain wheat is an awesome ingredient to appear first because it's part of a healthy meal plan. Avoid foods with ingredients like hydrogenated oil or partially hydrogenated oil, which are trans fats.

Putting the information to work

You might try choosing one section of the food label to focus on at first when shopping and evaluating products. You could also look at the food labels in your pantry at home to get familiar with the layout and information before you head to the store. You find out more about meal planning and grocery shopping in Chapter 12.

A food label may not make or break your purchase, but it may make you stop to think about whether you really want to drink an entire bottle of a smoothie to feel sated.

One of the most helpful things about food labels is that they allow you to compare and contrast foods. By looking at food labels, you can see whether one jar of pasta sauce has more sodium than another. You can make educated decisions. As consumers, this is the ticket to making healthy choices.

A Little Salt Goes a Long Way

Sodium, the main ingredient in salt, can increase your blood pressure. People with diabetes need to be cautious about high blood pressure because it can increase the risk of cardiovascular, eye, and kidney disease.

Therefore, eating less salt can lower your blood pressure.

The American Diabetes Association recommends less than 2,300 mg (1 teaspoon) of sodium a day, which is the same recommendation for people without diabetes. Talk with your dietitian about your sodium goals.

Most people eat way too much salt. Why? It's not that they're carrying around shakers of salt in their pockets. It's because many foods we eat (in packages or from restaurants) are loaded with sodium but don't taste salty.

Cheese, salad dressing, deli meat, canned soup, and tomato sauce commonly have high salt. Lots of other foods have high salt, too. Reading food labels is the only way to tell how much sodium is in foods you buy. Look at the milligrams (mg) and percent daily value of sodium to determine whether you should avoid certain foods.

VITAMINS AND SUPPLEMENTS: MAYBE NOT

The best way to get vitamins and minerals is by eating balanced meals from a variety of food groups. You don't need to take vitamins or other supplements unless your health-care provider recommends them.

Studies have shown that supplements such as chromium, magnesium, and vitamin D don't improve blood glucose. Neither do herbal supplements or remedies such as cinnamon.

The American Diabetes Association does not recommend that people with diabetes take fish oil supplements or other omega-3 supplements to boost their omega-3 levels. Instead, try to eat fish twice a week or find other sources such as walnuts and flaxseeds.

Satisfying Your Thirst

Food isn't the only thing you have to pay attention to when it comes to nutrition. Drinks run the gamut of good to bad, just as foods do. Of course, it's a good idea to pick the healthiest beverage (water) when you're thirsty. But that's not to say that you can't enjoy less healthy beverages every once in a while.

Drinking water, soda, and other beverages

If you're thirsty, drinking water is the best choice. Water is refreshing. Water is cheap. Water doesn't have calories. Water doesn't have added sugars or sodium. It's truly amazing.

You may have to make a concerted effort to drink water if it's not part of your normal routine. Keep a water bottle at your desk at work and one in your gym bag. Water bottles come in beautiful colors and fabulous designs to make carrying and drinking from them more fun.

The tap is the most abundant source of water in America. Yet, that shouldn't stop you from trying different kinds like sparkling water. The bubbles in San Pellegrino or Perrier may keep you drinking.

Drink flavored waters or fitness waters in moderation because they may contain added sugars, sodium, and other ingredients. Always check the label to see which nutrients and ingredients are included.

If you like some flavor in your water, add a slice of lemon, lime, or orange. How about raspberries or mint if you're feeling bold?

Plain coffee and tea can also be part of a healthy meal plan. Some studies have shown a benefit in drinking coffee to prevent type 2 diabetes; other studies have not. Enjoy your cup of joe in moderation, just like any other food or drink. Try to avoid adding cream, sugar, syrups, or flavors because they may have added sugars and excess calories.

Drinking a glass of low-fat or fat-free milk can also be a nutritious quencher. Try to avoid fruit and vegetable juices with added sugars or lots of sodium.

WARNING

Too much soda is bad for your health because it has added sugars. Limit added sugars because, in addition to affecting your blood glucose levels, they fill you up and can deter you from eating nutritious foods. Try to drink water instead of soda.

TIP

The American Diabetes Association recommends that people with type 2 diabetes drink sugar-free and calorie-free drinks including water and unsweetened coffee and tea.

Enjoying wine, beer, and spirits

Many people can safely drink wine, beer, and liquor if they have type 2 diabetes.

REMEMBER

Talk to your provider about whether alcohol is safe to drink with your existing medications and any other considerations. Women may be able to enjoy one or fewer alcoholic drinks per day, and men may be able to enjoy two or fewer alcoholic drinks per day. These are the same recommendations for people without diabetes. A drink is 12 ounces of beer, 5 ounces of wine, or 1½ ounces of spirits.

Keep in mind that alcohol can lower blood glucose, so it's important that people with diabetes not drink on an empty stomach, particularly those taking certain medications. Check your blood glucose if you're concerned — especially if you drink before you go to bed. Alcohol can lower blood glucose for up to 12 hours, so make sure you're not low before you fall asleep. The symptoms for low blood glucose can mimic the effects of intoxication, so always test your blood glucose if there's any concern. Be prepared by knowing the Rule of 15 and be ready to treat episodes of low blood glucose with glucose tablets or gels.

No one should drink and drive, and people with diabetes may want to be particularly vigilant about this safety rule. That's because people with diabetes may be more susceptible to episodes of low blood glucose, which combined with driving, can be dangerous for everyone on the road.

Alcohol also has calories, so talk to your dietitian about how to incorporate alcoholic drinks into your meal plans. People sometimes get hungry when drinking or have less self-control, so have a plan for not overindulging in unhealthy foods or giant portions. Mixers and premixed specialty drinks at the bar sometimes have lots of calories. Consider switching to no-calorie mixers like club soda or diet soda.

IN THIS CHAPTER

» **Choosing wholesome, nutritious foods**

» **Eyeballing ideal portion sizes**

» **Using a meal plan**

» **Getting familiar with carbohydrate counting**

» **Taking time to plan, shop, and cook**

» **Snacking, eating out, and celebrating special occasions**

Chapter **12**

Planning Healthy Meals

H ere's the fun part: After you know the basics of food and nutrition (refer to Chapter 11), it's time to use that knowledge to cook and enjoy delicious, healthy meals!

Delicious really is the focus. Plan meals you're passionate about and you can savor with every bite. You don't have to scrimp on flavor or feeling satisfied because you're using healthy ingredients.

Healthy eating for people with diabetes is the same as healthy eating for everyone. There's no such thing as a "diabetes diet." Instead, create your own meals based on your goals, lifestyle, and culture.

In this chapter, you discover three components of healthy eating: choosing a variety of wholesome foods, consuming healthy portions, and creating a meal plan that works for you. You also find out about carbohydrate counting and other eating plans commonly used by people with diabetes.

We also give you tips on how to plan meals, shop for ingredients, and cook healthy meals for yourself and your family. You find tips for snacking and eating out, as well as celebrating special occasions with confidence.

Considering Your Goals

Your goals are specific to you, so consider them thoughtfully as you embark on your journey of living with diabetes. Do you want to change how you look or feel? Do you want to live longer? Do you want to prevent certain diseases?

Working with a nutrition professional such as a registered dietitian can help you set realistic goals. It can be difficult to change behaviors and eating patterns on your own. You're going to benefit from support.

TIP

Your most valuable asset in devising healthy meals is your dietitian. He or she will assess your nutritional needs and help you personalize meals to fit your life and goals. Your dietitian can also be a certified diabetes educator (CDE). See Chapter 11 for more information on dietitians, including what they do, when to see one, and how to find out whether your insurance company will cover the cost of working with a dietitian.

People with type 2 diabetes often share common goals for healthy eating, as shown in the following list. You may want to do one of these things or all of them.

>> Keep A1C lower than 7.

>> Lower blood pressure to less than 140/90 mmHg.

>> Lower bad cholesterol (LDL) and triglycerides and boost your good cholesterol (HDL).

>> Lose or maintain weight.

>> Delay or prevent complications from diabetes.

The good news: Healthy eating can help you achieve these goals! It's not the only thing, though. Exercise, taking medications, and seeing your doctor are other important pieces.

REMEMBER

Exercise goes hand in hand with healthy eating. Eating well and exercising are the perfect pair for taking care of your diabetes — and helping you look and feel good. You find out more about exercise in Chapter 13, but keep it on your radar as you consider your goals.

Eating a Variety of Wholesome, Nutritious Foods

One component of healthy eating is choosing a variety of wholesome, nutritious foods. Well, that sounds okay, but what does that mean?

It means choosing foods that are more nutritious instead of foods that are less nutritious. Nutritious foods are low in saturated fats, added sugars, and refined grains.

The quality of your food matters, too. Choosing fish high in omega-3s such as salmon could improve your heart health. Choosing dark, leafy greens including kale, which is high in vitamins A, C, and K, could boost your immune system with its jolt of antioxidants.

Forget about a diabetes diet

There is no such thing as a diabetes diet. Yep, you heard it here. You won't find one diet that works for everyone with diabetes. You won't find a dietitian who prescribes one diet for all her patients with diabetes. You won't find a list of foods that fit into a prescribed diabetes plan.

Instead, it's up to you to choose foods that fit your goals, lifestyle, and culture. Sound daunting? Or liberating? Or perhaps a little of both.

On the bright side, it's wonderful to have choices (lots of choices). You don't have to deny yourself your favorite foods like chocolate cake or cheeseburgers if you have diabetes. It's less about denial and more about moderation.

If you love collard greens, you can find a recipe that helps you prepare them so you can eat them every week. If you adore cheese, you can choose low-fat varieties in small portions that you can eat every day. If you savor spicy chicken tikka masala, you can find a cookbook to help you tweak the ingredients to ramp up the flavor with less saturated fat.

Expanding the selection of foods you eat

REMEMBER

Being diagnosed with diabetes shouldn't feel like you're suddenly restricted to eating certain foods. Instead, you have the food world at your doorstep. You have the flexibility to choose foods that you truly enjoy from a variety of different plants and animals. You may discover and taste new foods you've never tried before.

Nutritious foods include almost every vegetable that you can think of under the sun. Nonstarchy vegetables are an easy choice because they're full of vitamins, minerals, and fiber, but with almost no calories. Arugula, broccoli, Brussels sprouts, mushrooms, and summer squash, not to mention fresh spinach and bell peppers, can be on your grocery list.

Fruits are nutritious, especially ones that you eat fresh without any sauces or sugar. Savor fruits in moderation so the natural sugars in these foods don't raise your blood glucose too much.

Whole grains such as oatmeal, whole-grain bread, whole-grain pastas, quinoa, and farro can't be beat for fiber, protein, and essential vitamins and minerals. They can protect against cardiovascular disease.

Nuts and seeds are chock-full of protein, fiber, vitamins, and healthy fats. Pecans, pistachios, pumpkin seeds, sesame seeds, almonds, and flaxseeds are just a handful of these tiny powerhouse players.

TIP

When planning your meals (more on that in a bit), do your best to choose foods from several of these categories each day. Doing so will ensure you get a variety of nutrients that your body needs to stay healthy.

If you need some help choosing the right foods, consider these excellent choices:

» Beans of any kind (kidney, pinto, black) are high in fiber, magnesium, and potassium.

» Dark green leafy vegetables like spinach, collards, and kale have vitamins and minerals and not many carbohydrates.

» Citrus fruits of all types (grapefruit, oranges, lemons, and limes) have fiber, vitamin C, and, most importantly, zest!

» Sweet potatoes are a starchy vegetable with fiber and vitamin A that you can try in place of white potatoes.

» Berries of any kind, including strawberries and blueberries, have fiber, vitamins, and antioxidants.

» Tomatoes have vitamins C and E and iron, and you can enjoy them so many ways: raw in salads, in sauces, or on your pizza.

» Fish high in omega-3 fats such as salmon, albacore tuna, and mackerel help reduce the risk of cardiovascular disease.

» Whole grains without any processing, such as barley, quinoa, and farro, are excellent sources of magnesium, chromium, proteins, fiber, and folate.

>> Walnuts and flaxseeds have omega-3 fats, and most nuts have protein, fiber, healthy fats, and vitamins and minerals.

>> Milk and yogurt are tried and true favorites for calcium and vitamin D.

Dishing Up Ideal Portions

You can eat a variety of healthy, wholesome foods (see the preceding section), but if you eat too much, you're not doing yourself any favors. Portions may seem like a mundane topic, but knowing the right portions for you is a powerful tool for eating well and maintaining or even losing weight.

Portion control can be one of the hardest things to do or perhaps learn, because your brain may already be preprogrammed. All-you-can-eat buffets are in business for a reason, after all.

You can change the way you think about portions, though. It may not come easily at first, so be patient with yourself as you practice. Ask your dietitian about tips for incorporating the right portion sizes for you into your meal plans (see Chapter 11 for more about working with a dietitian). How much an individual should eat is based on gender, age, height, weight goals, what else the person is eating, and the person's individual needs.

On a positive note, portion control can help you enjoy a variety of foods that you love. Perhaps nothing is totally off limits. Instead, you may choose to eat smaller portions of foods that are less healthy, such as sweets and fried foods.

Portion size and serving size are two different things. A *portion* is the amount of a particular food that you eat. It could be the cheeseburger that you order for lunch or the amount of tuna noodle casserole you spoon onto your plate. For example, average portion sizes have increased recently. We expect to eat more than we ever have in the past. A *serving size* is a measurement of food calculated by the U.S. Food and Drug Administration (FDA). Usually, you find serving sizes on food labels, but you may begin to use serving sizes as part of a meal plan. Serving sizes can help you eat a variety of foods, in the right amounts, throughout the day and calculate the amount of nutrients you're eating.

TIP

Portions and serving sizes may not add up. Sometimes, a portion size is larger than a serving size. For example, a foot-long sandwich portion from the sandwich shop may contain several servings of bread or meat.

By law, serving size is based on what people actually eat, instead of what they should eat. In 1993, the FDA created the Nutrition Facts label, which includes serving sizes that drew on certain standards called the *reference amounts customarily consumed* (RACCs). Since then, the RACCs have been revised to reflect Americans' increasing serving sizes of everything from ice cream to soda to muffins.

TIP

One way to enjoy even small portions of food is to savor each and every bite. If you're really looking forward to a bowl of ice cream as a treat, don't rush it. Take your time. Eat small bites. Focus on the flavor. Don't watch TV or look at your phone while you eat.

You can also look online for resources about serving sizes. Here are some more details about serving sizes for different foods.

Knowing what counts as one serving

According to the USDA, Each of the following counts as one serving:

>> 1 slice of bread

>> ½ cup cooked rice or pasta

>> 1 cup raw leafy vegetables

>> ½ cup other vegetables (raw or cooked)

>> 1 cup (8 ounces) milk

>> 1½ ounces cheese

>> 2–3 ounces of cooked meat, poultry, or fish

>> ⅓ cup nuts or 1 ounce

>> 2 tablespoons peanut butter

Weighing and measuring food

Weighing or measuring your food at home may be the best way to teach yourself about serving sizes and, therefore, your ideal portion. It takes practice to know what certain weights and amounts of food look like on your plate. As you practice, you'll be able to better gauge the right portion for you when you're at a restaurant or serving yourself fruit salad at a summer barbecue.

Using a scale is the most precise way to measure the amounts of food you're eating. Pastry chefs use kitchen scales all the time to weigh flour or sugar because it's so precise — and precision is everything when you're making soufflé. (Scales can be fun, too.)

TIP

If it's in your budget, buy a basic, cheap kitchen scale that you can use to measure foods as you prepare them at home. You can compare your usual portion to the serving size on the label to get a better idea of how much you're actually eating.

Measuring cups and spoons can be just as useful for figuring out an ideal portion or the number of servings. Serve yourself your usual portion of food. Now measure it using your scale or measuring cups. Is it more or fewer servings than you expected?

Here's an example: Two tablespoons of peanut butter is one serving. Measure out 2 tablespoons before you spread it on your toast in the morning. It's the best way to determine whether you actually consume one serving size.

Knowing how to create your plate

Some people find the plate method, also called Create Your Plate, a simple and effective way to plan portions and eat healthy foods. It may also help you manage your blood glucose and lose weight.

Create Your Plate is a straightforward strategy where you envision dividing your plate into sections and filling each section with a different group of food (see Figure 12-1). You can still choose the foods you want, but you serve yourself those foods in specific portions.

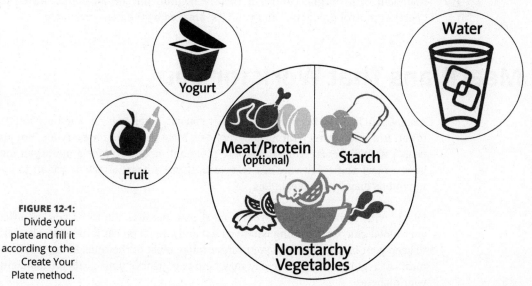

FIGURE 12-1:
Divide your plate and fill it according to the Create Your Plate method.

Courtesy of the American Diabetes Association

The advantage of Create Your Plate is that you don't need any special tools. You can use it at home, at a restaurant during lunch, or at a potluck in your neighborhood.

Here are the steps to follow to Create Your Plate:

1. **Using your dinner plate, envision a line down the middle of the plate. Then on one side, divide it again so you have three sections on your plate.**

2. **Fill the largest section with nonstarchy vegetables like broccoli, arugula, tomatoes, asparagus, and mushrooms.**

3. **Now in one of the small sections, put grains and starchy foods, such as whole-grain pasta or sweet potatoes.**

4. **In the other small section, put your protein such as chicken, fish, or pork.**

5. **Consider whether you plan to eat a serving of fruit, milk, or yogurt because they have carbohydrates and might impact your choices in Step 3.**

6. **Choose healthy fats in small amounts.**

   For cooking, use oils. For salads, some healthy additions are nuts, seeds, avocado, and vinaigrettes.

7. **To complete your meal, add a zero-calorie drink like water, unsweetened tea, or coffee.**

TIP

You can buy specialty plates, measuring containers, lunch boxes, and other tools that help with portion control if they're helpful. Just do an online search for "portion control products," and you'll be amazed by the items available.

Meal Plans That Work for You

A meal plan is just a fancy name for what you eat, when you eat, and how you like to eat. It's your strategy for meals every day. Meal plans are for everyone, not just people with diabetes. Women who are pregnant or training for a marathon may have a meal plan. Men who are recovering from a heart attack or trying to lose 10 pounds may have a meal plan.

People with diabetes benefit from a meal plan because the foods you eat affect your blood glucose. Planning what you eat and when you eat it can make it easier to keep your blood glucose in your target range most of the time. Eating healthful meals at regular times of the day may help you achieve your goals for managing your diabetes.

REMEMBER

Keeping blood glucose in your target range can help you feel good each day, and also reduce the risk of complications like heart, eye, and kidney disease as you get older. It may help you achieve your goals of maintaining or losing weight, too.

Try not to look at a meal plan as a diet. It's not. Diets are usually considered short-term fixes that restrict foods. Diets can make you hungry. Diets aren't sustainable for the rest of your life. Diets aren't usually fun.

A meal plan is a way to build the foods that you adore into your life. You can choose wholesome, nutritious flavors that you truly enjoy. Think about portion size, too (see the earlier section "Dishing Up Ideal Portions").

Forget about a diabetes meal plan

Just as there is no diabetes diet (see the "Forget about a diabetes diet" earlier in this chapter), there is no diabetes meal plan. People with diabetes use different meal plans to achieve their goals. The critical thing is to meet with a dietitian so you can create a meal plan that works for you.

A meal plan helps you come up with strategies for what you eat: breakfast, lunch, dinner, and snacks. It gives you guidelines for when you eat your meals, like eating breakfast as soon as you hop out of bed in the morning or eating dinner at least 3 hours before you go to bed.

REMEMBER

A meal plan is adaptable. It's not set in stone and should allow you the flexibility to enjoy special occasions like eating dinner out for birthdays or enjoying an extra snack because you walked 3 miles. Additionally, a meal plan can change over time based on your goals, lifestyle, or health.

The most important component of a meal plan is you. A meal plan must fit you. What does that mean? A meal plan should reflect your diabetes or other health goals, lifestyle, and culture. If it doesn't, you probably won't follow it. Or you'll try your best to follow it for a few months, but then go back to your usual eating habits.

Turning to a dietitian for help

Schedule an appointment with a dietitian so you can develop a meal plan together. Your dietitian will evaluate your preferences, nutritional needs, and your health, including your diabetes. Then the two of you can discuss the options for creating a healthy eating plan.

TIP

Try not to think of your diabetes meal plan as static. It may evolve and change as your goals and lifestyle change. You'll probably need to refresh it — on your own or with your dietitian — to make sure it's working for you.

It's a good idea to see a dietitian when you're first diagnosed with diabetes or soon after. Then, if you can, make an appointment with a dietitian at least yearly for a refresh. (See Chapter 11 for more details on dietitians, nutrition appointments, and insurance coverage.)

Coming up with your own meal plan

If you don't have the time or resources to see a dietitian right now, you can come up with your own meal plan. In this section, you'll find descriptions of some of the most popular meal plans. For more information, visit www.diabetes.org or www.choosemyplate.gov, or ask your diabetes care provider or CDE for more information on meal planning.

If you're looking for a great place to start without too much preparation, check out a description of the Create Your Plate method earlier in this chapter. Ask your physician or healthcare provider whether this is the right approach for you.

Mediterranean-style eating plan

The Mediterranean-style eating plan has been touted as a good plan for people with diabetes. The name comes from how traditional people living near the Mediterranean Sea in places like Italy and Greece typically eat. These people live long, healthy lives.

TECHNICAL STUFF

It's sometimes called the "Mediterranean diet," but it's also called the Mediterranean-style eating plan because it's truly a style and way of eating.

In general, following a Mediterranean-style eating plan means eating fresh vegetables and fruits, whole grains and nuts, and small amounts of fish and chicken. Cook with olive oil instead of butter, and enjoy a glass of red wine.

Most people choose a Mediterranean-style eating plan because of its health benefits, particularly for preventing heart disease and stroke. Also, the Mediterranean-style eating plan is a good alternative to a low-fat diet for reducing the risk of type 2 diabetes.

In people with diabetes, a Mediterranean-style eating plan can reduce A1C. Also, studies have shown that the Mediterranean-style eating plan can improve cholesterol and other risk factors for cardiovascular disease in people with diabetes. The American Diabetes Association doesn't recommend any specific meal plan for all people with diabetes, but consider it as one of many options for healthy eating.

Perhaps you just want to incorporate the parts you like best out of the Mediterranean-style eating plan, like enjoying fresh fruits and vegetables in season. You may want to use olive oil or other healthy fats when cooking or making salad dressings.

TIP

It doesn't have to be an all-or-nothing approach, although some people may enjoy the structure of following a cohesive approach to eating. What follows are tips for Mediterranean-style eating:

>> Enjoy your food, and make healthful eating a family affair. For example, cook and eat with your friends and family, and make sure you sit down and enjoy your food with others.

>> Include plants, such as seasonal fresh vegetables and fruits, as a majority of the food choices in your day.

>> Use herbs and spices to season your foods so you have flavor without added salt, sugar, and butter.

>> Use olive oil for cooking, instead of saturated fats like butter.

>> Beans, nuts, legumes, and whole grains are everyday staples and great sources of wholesome carbohydrate and protein.

>> Eat lean proteins such as chicken, low-fat dairy, eggs, and cheese, and enjoy fish twice a week.

>> Enjoy occasional desserts in small portions and choose fruits often.

>> Sip a glass of wine with your meal, and drink lots of water throughout the day.

>> Stay active throughout the day by taking frequent breaks from sitting. Bike and walk to work or to the grocery store.

Food choices/exchanges

Following a meal plan based on food choices/exchanges may be a good option if you want more precision than the plate method, but don't want to count each carbohydrate (see more about carb counting in the following sections). Food choices used to be called food exchanges, but you may still hear both terms.

Food choices/exchanges are used to describe a certain quantity of food within each *food list* (a grouping of foods with similar nutrient profiles). For example, a small piece of fresh fruit is one Fruit choice and ⅓ cup of cooked pasta is one Starch choice. Meet with a dietitian to plan how many food choices from each food list you'll eat at meals or during a day.

The American Diabetes Association publishes a booklet of food lists — *Choose Your Foods: Food Lists for Diabetes*, which is co-published by the Academy of Nutrition and Dietetics — for people who use food choices/exchanges to plan their meals. This booklet can be bought online at www.shopdiabetes.org.

Low-carb meal plans

Following a low-carb meal plan is a popular strategy for people with diabetes. There isn't one single low-carb plan, however; there are hundreds.

In general, with a low-carb plan, the focus is on eating protein such as beef, poultry, fish, eggs, and nuts. You eat vegetables low in carbohydrates such as leafy greens, cucumbers, and broccoli. And you try to avoid added sugars and grain products such as pasta, rice, and bread.

Studies are inconclusive about the health benefits of low-carb meal plans for people with diabetes. Some studies show benefits in terms of blood glucose and risk of cardiovascular disease. Other studies show that higher-carb diets are beneficial. The jury is still out.

The American Diabetes Association doesn't recommend or discourage a low-carb meal plan. Instead, you should consider it as one of many options for healthy eating. Talk with your dietitian about the best plan for you.

REMEMBER

Following a low-carb meal plan may be a good option for some people with diabetes, depending on their needs. But it's important to note that no one, including people with diabetes, should try to eliminate carbs from his diet completely, even though carbs have the biggest impact on blood glucose levels. Carbohydrates provide energy that helps the body and brain to function properly.

TECHNICAL STUFF

Some consider the paleo diet a low-carb meal plan because the two eating styles share many common elements. A paleo diet is based on the concept that people should eat like humans during the Stone Age or Paleolithic Period before farming was widespread. With a paleo diet you eat vegetables, fruits, nuts, seeds, lean meats, and fish. You avoid grains, dairy products, refined sugar, salt, potatoes, and highly refined foods. You drink a lot of water and exercise regularly. The American Diabetes Association doesn't recommend or discourage a paleo diet, so talk with your dietitian if you're considering it.

TECHNICAL STUFF

Scientists continue to study the effects of low-carb diets on people with diabetes. For example, one review of studies that examined low-carb versus high-carb diets found no difference in terms of blood glucose management in people with type 2 diabetes. In fact, the total number of calories that you eat appears more important than where you get them in terms of carbohydrates or proteins. Talk to your dietitian or healthcare provider to determine the best meal plan for you.

Intro to Carbohydrate Counting

Carbohydrate counting is another strategy that you can use to plan your meals. It means focusing on carbohydrates as you think about when and how much to eat. With carbohydrate counting, your meal plan includes eating a certain number of carbohydrates or servings of carbohydrates each meal or snack. One carbohydrate serving is equal to 15 grams of carbohydrate.

REMEMBER

Carbohydrates are a big deal. They're the main source of energy in your body, in addition to protein and fat. When eaten, carbohydrates break down into smaller sugars, including glucose, which the cells convert into energy for the body. Carbohydrates provide fuel for the central nervous system and the brain. (For more on carbohydrates, flip back to Chapter 11.)

Counting and eating a planned amount of carbohydrates can help keep your blood glucose in your target range. The American Diabetes Association does not have recommendations regarding the amount of carbohydrates that people with type 2 diabetes should eat each day. Instead, eat carbohydrates in moderation just like other nutrients such as protein and fat.

Balance carbohydrates with other foods such as nonstarchy vegetables, protein, and healthy fats.

TIP

If you're interested in carbohydrate counting, talk to your dietitian about coming up with a personalized plan for how many carbohydrates will work for you at meals and snacks. We give you an introduction here, but we encourage you to bring up it up with your dietitian or CDE so you can get more specifics for your situation. Your dietitian can take into account your preferences and what you have been eating, your weight, activity levels, medications, and goals for blood glucose.

Calling out carbohydrates

Certain foods are high in carbohydrates, and they may affect your blood glucose much more than other foods. Meats, nonstarchy vegetables, and fats have less of an effect on blood glucose. Check out this partial list of foods that contain carbohydrates:

» Bread, bagels, biscuits, muffins, and tortillas

» Boxed and ready-to-eat cereal

» Pasta and couscous

» Rice

- ❯❯ Cornmeal and grits

- ❯❯ Starchy vegetables such as corn, peas, potatoes, and sweet potatoes

- ❯❯ Pancakes and waffles

- ❯❯ Popcorn, potato chips, pretzels, and rice cakes

- ❯❯ Beans (such as kidney, black, garbanzo, lima, and pinto) and lentils

- ❯❯ Fruit and fruit juice

- ❯❯ Milk, soymilk, and yogurt

- ❯❯ Sugar, such as table sugar or syrup

- ❯❯ Sweets such as candy, cookies, doughnuts, ice cream, frozen yogurt, honey, jam and jelly, cake, pie, and pudding

Portion matters

Portion and serving sizes matter with carbohydrates, too. Eating a huge bowl of pasta raises your blood glucose more than eating a side of pasta with your salad and grilled chicken. Everyone has seen those gigantic apples at the grocery store (they're probably not one serving size, right?).

If you're interested in carbohydrate counting, you may want to invest in a scale or measuring cups so you can start to visualize serving sizes better. (See the "Weighing and measuring food" section earlier in this chapter.)

TIP

You can download an app that helps you estimate, record, and track your carbohydrates. Search iTunes or Google Play for highly rated and popular carbohydrate counting apps.

Reading food labels for carbohydrates

A food label is a fabulous resource for learning how many carbohydrates are in your foods (for more on reading food labels, see Chapter 11). First, if you're counting carbohydrates, then you'll want to focus on the grams (not percent daily value).

Next, look for the "Total Carbohydrate" line. It will tell you how many grams of carbohydrates are in one serving.

Look at the line underneath Total Carbohydrate called "Dietary Fiber." Dietary Fiber is included in the amount of Total Carbohydrate (that's why it's smaller and underneath). Dietary Fiber is a type of carbohydrate that is either partially digested or not digested, so it may have less of an impact on your blood glucose than other types of carbohydrate like sugar. Fiber helps with digestive health, and all adults should aim to eat 25–30 grams of carbohydrate per day. If you use insulin, ask your dietitian or diabetes care provider whether and how eating foods with a lot of fiber will impact your insulin needs.

Now, examine the next line underneath called "Sugars." Sugars are included in the amount of Total Carbohydrate (that's why it's small and underneath, just like fiber). Remember that the grams of Total Carbohydrate, not Dietary Fiber or Sugars, are what you track when counting carbohydrates. Are you planning to eat just one serving or the whole container? You'll need to check the servings per container next to see whether your package has one or more servings. Then check the serving size to determine how many servings you plan to eat.

For example, say you want 15 grams of carbohydrate for a snack. Your box of crackers has 15 grams of Total Carbohydrate per serving, but there are two servings per container. The serving size is 1 ounce, or about 18 crackers, so you'd only eat half the box or 18 crackers to get 15 grams of carbohydrate.

TECHNICAL STUFF

INVESTIGATING THE GLYCEMIC INDEX

You may hear the terms *glycemic index* or *glycemic load* to refer to certain foods or meal plans.

Glycemic index is a ranking of carbohydrate-containing foods, based on the food's effect on blood glucose levels compared with a standard reference food (such as pure glucose).

Glycemic load is a measurement of the impact that the carbohydrate in a certain food or meal has on blood glucose levels. It is calculated by multiplying a food's glycemic index by its amount of carbohydrate. Food items are designated as having a low, medium, or high glycemic load. Glycemic load is mostly used in research studies and is probably not a practical tool for most people with diabetes to use for everyday meal planning.

The American Diabetes Association does not endorse or discourage specific meal plans based on the glycemic index or glycemic load. Ask your dietitian or diabetes care provider if you have questions about these terms.

Planning, Shopping, and Cooking Smart

After you've chosen a healthy meal plan, the fun begins. Now you get to prepare and eat scrumptious foods!

Planning, shopping, and cooking for yourself and your family can be one of the most fulfilling things that you do in your day. It's a real joy for some people. But like most of us today, you may feel like you don't have the time. Don't worry. In this section, we give you some tips for saving time and making steps easier.

If you don't have much experience in the kitchen or don't really enjoy cooking, the good news is you don't have to do everything at once. Maybe start by making one home-cooked meal a week or every two weeks and gradually work your way up to more.

This is not a comprehensive list of strategies. After all, entire books cover the topic of healthy cooking with diabetes. If you're interested in more tips and information, go to www.shopdiabetes.org to find terrific books on this topic.

Planning smart

Before you can shop for and cook meals, you need a plan. Carve out time to think about what you'd like to eat for the week. This could be on your commute home from work or when you're walking the dog in the evening.

Come up with a plan for the week, including breakfasts, lunches, dinners, and snacks (if you can). Consider your schedule and time constraints on certain days so you don't overcommit yourself.

Seek out and select recipes ahead of time. Look for inspiration everywhere: magazines, cookbooks, online, your best friend. Rip pages out of magazines, dog-ear cookbooks, or find an app that saves your online recipes.

As you plan your meals and select recipes, consider your goals. When considering a recipe, look at the total amount of calories and carbohydrate in a serving size. And look at the serving size. Will this fit with your goals? Check out other factors or nutrients that may be important to you. For example, maybe you're trying to reduce saturated fat and sodium in your meal plan. Or maybe one of your goals is to include more omega-3 fats in your meals to boost your heart health; in that case, look for recipes with ingredients rich in omega-3 fats.

Or let's say you're counting carbohydrates and you want to eat 30 grams of carbohydrates per meal. In that case, you probably shouldn't plan a meal that includes pasta, garlic bread, and a dessert. Instead, look at the recipe or nutrition label of the foods you're considering, and count up the number of carbohydrates per ingredient or food. You may need to skip the garlic bread and/or dessert and instead have a leafy green salad with your pasta.

Before you head out to the grocery store, write down all the ingredients you'll need on paper or use an app on your phone to record them. That way you won't forget anything, and it will make shopping faster and easier.

Consider stocking your pantry with healthy, essential ingredients so you have them on hand when you don't have time to shop. These items might include olive oil, whole-wheat pasta, beans, garlic, onions, brown rice, canned vegetables, and canned tuna in water.

TIP
You can find a bounty of recipes on the American Diabetes Association website (www.diabetes.org) or in American Diabetes Association cookbooks like *Quick Diabetic Recipes For Dummies* (Wiley) or others available from www.shopdiabetes.org.

Plan for snacks to have on hand, and write down those ingredients, too. See more on savvy snacking later in this chapter.

Shopping smart

You've heard this before, but it's true: Don't shop when you're hungry. You're more likely to buy unhealthy snacks and food you don't need.

Use your list to shop for only necessary ingredients. Try to buy the majority of your foods from the fresh vegetable and fruits section instead of the packaged-food aisles. It's one way to avoid added sugars and saturated fats.

Really look at the produce. Which looks the tastiest, freshest, and most in season? Use all your senses, including your nose to smell and hands to feel for the best fruits and vegetables. You're more likely to eat something that looks and smells delicious. Also, seasonal produce may be less expensive or on sale, versus produce that is out of season.

TIP
Don't be afraid to use the scale in the produce section. It's there for a reason: you. Find out how many ounces are in the apple you want to buy or how many heads of broccoli you need for your recipe.

If you do need to pick up some packaged foods, like pasta or bread, make sure to check out the food labels. Compare a couple of different brands to see how the food's nutrients compare. Remember to look at the serving size when thinking about how much you'll eat. It's very important. Then look at the number of calories per serving to see whether it fits into your total calorie goal for the day (if you have one). Consider the total carbohydrates as you think about eating a variety of foods such as carbohydrates, proteins, and lots of nonstarchy vegetables. You may be surprised to find a low-fat food is higher in carbohydrates than a full-fat food is. Balance your goals for carbohydrates with your goals for reducing saturated fats.

Cooking smart

If you have time when you get home from the store, try to wash and dry your produce so it's ready to use for cooking. It's easier and quicker to make a salad when the lettuce is already washed and dried.

Consider chopping up some of the vegetables and storing them in little baggies or containers, making them easy to dump in the pan for your recipe or grab for a snack. It's quicker to grab a healthy vegetable for a snack when it's prepared instead of having to wash, peel, and slice it in the moment. However, washed and prepared vegetables may not last as long, so balance these considerations.

Try baking and grilling foods if you normally fry them. Use healthy fats such as olive oil, avocado oil, sesame oil, canola oil, and others to sauté foods or make salad dressings. Try to avoid cooking with butter or lard.

Spices and herbs are your secret to flavorful, robust foods without added fat or sugar. Use them instead of extra salt to get the best taste sensations out of your foods. Salt-free spice mixtures are one option. Try fresh herbs like parsley, basil, rosemary, and cilantro.

Zests of ingredients such as fresh lemon or ginger can also punch up your food without added calories.

Put on your favorite music while you cook for easy inspiration and motivation. It doesn't matter what genre; music can get your feet moving in the kitchen and can make cooking more fun.

Tempting Your Taste Buds with Nutritious Nibbles

Planning what you're going to eat for snacks is just as important as planning what you're going to eat during meals. In fact, healthy snacks can be part of your meal plan. Ask your dietitian or diabetes care provider whether including snacks in your meal plan is right for you.

Snacks aren't the enemy. They give you energy and curb hunger. They also raise your blood glucose if it's below your target range after exercising or if you've gone longer than usual between meals. See Chapter 8 for details on treating lows with the Rule of 15, which includes eating a food with 15 grams of carbohydrates.

If you're carbohydrate counting as part of your meal plan, you may want to think of your foods in terms of their carbohydrates and their ability to raise your blood glucose. This could be helpful if you need a quick burst of energy before working out or if you feel like your blood glucose is low.

Avoid snacks while you're watching TV or looking at your phone. This can lead to mindless snacking, and perhaps overeating. Savor and enjoy your snacks.

The amount of carbs to eat when snacking will vary for different people; the right amount for you will be based on your individual needs. Some people may need low-carb snacks; others may need 20–30 grams of carbohydrate (you may need a higher-carb snack before a strenuous workout, for example). Your dietitian can help you determine whether snacks are right for you, and how many grams of carbohydrate to eat at each snack. Here are some examples of healthy snacks with various amounts of carbs. These options are more nutritious alternatives to traditional snack foods such as candies, cookies, chips, pretzels, dips, and other sugary or starchy foods.

If you're looking for a relatively low-carb option, snacks with less than 5 grams of carbs include the following:

>> 1 ounce of nuts like almonds, pistachios, or peanuts

>> 5 baby carrots

>> A hard-boiled egg

>> 2 tablespoons of pumpkin or sesame seeds

>> 1 cup of light popcorn

>> 1 string cheese stick

>> 10 goldfish crackers

Snacks with a moderate amount of carbs (10–20 grams of carbs) include the following:

>> A small apple or orange

>> ⅓ cup of hummus and 1 cup of fresh veggies

>> ¼ cup of dried fruit and nut mix

>> ¼ cup of cottage cheese and ½ cup of fresh or canned fruit

If higher-carb snacks are right for you, munch on one of these snacks, which have about 30 grams of carbs:

>> A banana with 1 tablespoon of peanut butter

>> ¾ cup of whole-grain cereal with ½ cup of skim milk

>> 6 ounces of light yogurt and ¾ cup of blueberries, blackberries, or raspberries

Eating Out with Confidence

Eating out is a pleasure and treat. You can try foods that you never dreamed of whipping up in your kitchen. And it's often the go-to option for families or couples on busy weeknights when there just isn't time to cook.

However, eating out can be challenging for anyone and particularly people with diabetes because you have little control over ingredients. You might feel like you're at the mercy of the restaurant, so you just throw up your hands.

Don't despair. You can take steps to eat healthy foods while eating out. We've got you covered.

Selecting restaurants with healthy choices

It may seem like there is a fast-food restaurant on every corner. However, there are also healthy restaurant options. You just may have to do a bit of searching to find them.

Restaurants with healthy options run the gamut from fast food to sit down. The Internet may be your best resource for choosing a restaurant with healthy meals. Most restaurants post their menus on their websites, and some even have the nutritional values for each dish.

Look for menus that have a variety of salads or even dishes labeled "heart healthy." Sodium is everywhere when you eat out — from fast food to fine dining. Ask restaurants whether they have low-sodium options if you're concerned about reducing sodium.

Check out the book *Eat Out, Eat Well* by Hope Warshaw for more great tips on this subject (available from www.shopdiabetes.org).

Ordering meals that mesh with your plan

After you choose a restaurant that seems suitable for your needs and the occasion, stop and think ahead before it's time to order your meal. You may be tempted to throw the rules out the window for just one meal, but consider how you'll feel later. Instead, follow these tips to eat well and have an enjoyable experience:

» Ask your server whether nutritional information on dishes is available. Some restaurants, especially fast food, have these available. Read the nutritional information to make the best choice. Avoid dishes high in calories, saturated fats, or added sugars.

   If the restaurant doesn't have nutritional information on hand, ask about serving sizes and ingredients in dishes before you order.

» If you have the option, ask to have fish or meat baked or grilled instead of fried.

» To avoid salt, ask that salt be omitted or ask whether there are low-sodium options.

» Order salad dressings, sauces, or gravies on the side so you can control how much you eat.

» If the main entrees don't look healthy, consider ordering a salad, sharing your entrée, or saving half the entrée for later.

» Don't be shy about asking for substitutions like fresh vegetables instead of french fries.

» If your plate arrives and the portions are larger than you expected, ask for an extra plate or to-go container. Put the excess food in it to eat later.

» Don't supersize or order jumbo anything. These items tend to be high in saturated fat and calories. You've never seen a supersized carrot on the menu, have you?

» Just because you get a free soda with your meal deal, doesn't mean you have to fill your cup with soda. Fill it with ice water instead. You'll avoid added calories and sugar. The same goes for that bag of chips; you don't have to eat them now.

Celebrating Holidays and Special Occasions

People with diabetes may get most frustrated with their meal plan or eating choices during the holidays or on special occasions. Holidays especially are steeped in tradition and culture — and food. It can be hard to enjoy a holiday when everything seems to revolve around food that isn't often healthy.

Planning ahead is one key to success during the holidays or when celebrating special occasions. It will give you back control so you don't feel like you're just reacting to food.

Think about when meals are typically served. If you know that a big meal is served at night, you might consider that when making choices about food earlier in the day.

Choose smaller portions so you can try foods that you enjoy. Offer to bring a vegetable dish that you know is healthy to ensure an option that you can enjoy at the gathering.

Plan to get exercise during the holidays, which can lower your blood glucose and improve your mood. Focus on the positive choices that you can make, such as spending time with family and friends. You'll find more about emotional health and support in Chapter 14.

REMEMBER

If you get off track during the holidays, don't let it ruin your attitude. Just readjust. If you've overindulged, try to get back on track. If you need to go for a walk, put on your sneakers and head out the front door. Find someone who is a source of support to keep your spirits up.

TIP

Planning ahead to fit in your favorite dessert during the holidays or on your birthday can help keep your blood glucose in the target range, even if you have diabetes. You may just want to enjoy a smaller portion to stay within your meal plan. Ask your dietitian how to make accommodations for special foods or desserts.

IN THIS CHAPTER

» **Checking out all the benefits of exercise**

» **Getting up and moving**

» **Seeing your different exercise options**

» **Going through the routine**

» **Staying motivated**

Chapter **13**

Amping Up Your Exercise

E xercise is one of the best things you can do for your body and mind. When you have type 2 diabetes, exercise can affect your diabetes directly by lowering blood glucose and improving your body's sensitivity to insulin. And that's just the tip of the iceberg. Exercise has all sorts of amazing benefits, which we cover in this chapter.

Maybe you don't consider yourself an athlete or even a regular gym goer. Luckily, you don't have to be either to reap the benefits of regular physical activity. You can start small and choose activities you enjoy.

Exercise is not a one-size-fits-all activity. Not everyone wants to don spandex and hit a spin-cycling class every night. There are different types of exercise for people of different ages and physical abilities — not to mention different interests.

TIP

What's the difference between physical activity and exercise? Not much. Sometimes exercise is considered a subcategory or more structured form of physical activity. However, in this chapter and throughout the book, we use the terms interchangeably.

Keep the information from this chapter in mind as you start moving more often in your everyday life. Choose activities that you truly enjoy and that you can fit into your day.

In this chapter, we give you the tools to take these steps (both figuratively and literally). You get details about exercise benefits, what to do first, different types and stages of exercise, and motivators to keep you going.

If, after reading this chapter, you want more details about how exercise can help you control your diabetes or some guidance for creating a quality fitness program, check out *Diabetes & Keeping Fit For Dummies* by Dr. Sheri R. Colberg (Wiley).

1, 2, 3: Counting the Many Benefits of Exercise

The benefits of exercise are enormous — especially for people with type 2 diabetes. Exercise can lower blood glucose. When you exercise, your body uses glucose (stored as glycogen and released as glucose) in your muscles and liver for energy. Then as you deplete those stores, your muscles use glucose from your blood for energy (lowering blood glucose). Exercise can also make your muscles and other tissues more sensitive to insulin, which means your body uses insulin better. Physical activity benefits A1C, one of the main measurements of blood glucose control.

The effects of exercise are immediate. In one small study, people with type 2 diabetes who exercised for one session of high-intensity cycling improved their blood glucose for up to 24 hours.

TECHNICAL STUFF

In another study, an 8-week structured exercise program lowered A1C by 0.66 percent in people with type 2 diabetes. This benefit happened without changes in body mass index. In other words, exercise helped with blood glucose regardless of weight.

Exercise is also good for your blood vessels, and it can lower your risk for heart disease and stroke. It lowers blood pressure and improves blood lipids. It can help you lose or maintain your weight, which can improve both. For example, over time, aerobic exercise can benefit HDL (good) cholesterol and blood pressure.

Burning calories is one reason many people exercise. In Chapter 12, we talk about calories in (with food) and calories out (with physical activity). It's a simple equation. If you want to maintain your weight, you need to burn the same number of calories you eat. If you want to lose weight, you need to burn more calories than you eat. Exercising is the best way to reach these goals.

Exercise also helps you sleep better at night, and getting more shut-eye is something everyone can agree on. People who exercise report improvements in their quality and quantity of sleep.

METABOLISM AND WEIGHT

Perhaps you've heard people say, "I have a high metabolism — I don't gain a lot of weight," or "I wish I could speed up my metabolism — I'll never lose weight at this rate." So, how does metabolism affect your weight?

Metabolism is a complex process, but it's basically how your body turns the things you eat and drink into energy. If you eat and drink more than is required to fuel your body, your body stores that extra energy in the form of fat. Exercise is a way to break that cycle.

In addition to the amount of calories in (food) and calories out (exercise), your metabolism affects how many calories you burn. Scientists are still studying the complex factors that go into metabolism such as gender and genetics. One thing that we know for sure, as you get older, your metabolism slows. For example, when you're 60, you may have to work a little harder to lose weight than you did when you were 20. This means that exercise can be so beneficial as you get older, helping you burn calories and lose or maintain weight.

Mood and symptoms of depression can also be improved with exercise. Exercise changes your neural pathways in positive ways and releases feel-good brain chemicals called *endorphins.* It also helps distract you from daily worries and anxieties by focusing your energy on something different. This can help with stress, too!

Exercising regularly can also strengthen your muscles and bones so your body is stronger and less fragile. It can improve your balance and flexibility. That's not just important to your diabetes care but to your life in general. With a bit more exercise, you may soon be able to bend your knees to garden or chase after your grandson in the front yard or just exit your car more gracefully.

It's hard to argue with all the benefits of exercise.

Keep in mind that exercising and losing weight can also help prevent or delay type 2 diabetes. So, if you know someone at risk for type 2 diabetes, bring her along on your walk! She may benefit from some fresh air and physical activity, too! Plus, it's always more fun to exercise with a friend.

First Steps to Physical Activity

Getting active is easier than you think. It can be short, low-intensity bouts of daily activity. You don't have to move mountains every day. And if you're not in the habit of getting a lot of exercise, it's best to start out slowly and work your way up to longer and more-intense workouts.

For example, walking 10 minutes a day may be a doable first goal. You can build from there by adding extra minutes or by doing 10-minute walks two or three times a day.

The following sections offer ideas about adding physical activity to your day, explain what health issues to be on the lookout for, and give you some tips on setting fitness goals.

Sitting less and moving more

Everyone with diabetes (and even people without diabetes) should sit less and move more. In fact, this can be the first place you start with physical activity.

REMEMBER

The American Diabetes Association recommends that people with type 2 diabetes sit less. When you're sitting, get up every 30 minutes for 3–4 minutes of activity or standing to improve your blood glucose.

Moving more can include doing unstructured activities during the day such as walking the dog, cleaning the house, gardening, and turning off the TV to do something that requires you to get up and move.

Stand up more often and for longer periods. For example, when you're playing a game on your phone or texting, stand up instead of sitting on the couch.

Walk more, even fewer than 15 minutes, several times a day. Think of ways to take short walks at home or in the workplace: Head to the mailbox at the end of the driveway or to a bathroom located on a different floor of your office building.

If you want to do more than just stand up or walk around, try some of these easy exercises to get your muscles moving:

>> Leg lifts or extensions

>> Overhead arm stretches

>> Desk chair swivels

>> Torso twists

>> Side lunges

>> Walking in place

TIP

Incorporate fun into your physical activity. Take your kids to the park and push them on the swings, play Simon Says, fly a kite, or play an easy game of tag. By the end of the afternoon, you'll feel great about life and you'll forget that you were taking part in physical activity.

Sitting less and moving more is a way of life that everyone with type 2 diabetes should embrace. For those just starting out, these daily changes may be enough. But for the majority of people with type 2 diabetes, these daily changes should be in addition to more-structured exercise (see the "Considering Different Types of Exercise" section later in the chapter for details).

Talking to your healthcare provider

REMEMBER

Talk with your healthcare provider before you start an exercise routine or start exercising differently. Your physician can give you a checkup so you're both aware of any limitations or stressors.

Your physician may check your heart, blood vessels, cholesterol, and A1C before you begin. If you have complications of diabetes, such as nerve damage, kidney disease, or heart disease, your physician can tell you which types of exercise and what intensity levels are safe for you. In some cases, she may refer you to a specialist called an *exercise physiologist* (a specialist trained in the science of exercise who can help you plan a safe and effective exercise program).

Checking blood glucose during exercise

The great news about exercise is that it can lower your blood glucose, but it can also put some people at risk for hypoglycemia. Many people with type 2 diabetes don't need to worry about hypoglycemia during exercise. However, some people taking insulin or pills that stimulate insulin production (sulfonylureas and glinides) may experience lows during exercise, so they may need to check their blood glucose before and after exercise. Some providers may suggest reducing the amount of rapid-acting insulin if you're anticipating rigorous, prolonged exercise. Or it may be a good idea to carry a snack along during exercise if you take insulin or the above-mentioned pills.

TIP

Ask your physician what's right for you — and whether and when you should check your blood glucose during exercise. She may recommend that you check your blood glucose the first few times you try more-intense workouts so you have a better sense of how these workouts affect your body. After that, you may not need to check as regularly unless you're concerned about a low. Or she may recommend that you check before and after each workout and bring a snack.

Thinking about your fitness goals

Everyone exercises for different reasons, but most people with diabetes share common goals of lowering their A1C, losing weight, and destressing. Think about what you want to achieve so you can create personal and meaningful goals and find the motivation to get there. (For more about motivation and support, see the "Motivators to Keep You Going" section later in this chapter.)

Not every goal has to be related to your diabetes. You may have a goal of looking a certain way by your summer vacation at the beach. You may want to inspire others in your family to get active. Or you may hope to uncover newfound energy at the end of the day or on the weekends. Your goals are personal and meaningful, so don't disregard them.

Conceptualizing these goals will help you come up with a plan for exercise. After all, exercise should be convenient, doable, and enjoyable or it's not going to happen. You're the only one who knows what works best for your schedule, lifestyle, and goals.

TIP

When coming up with fitness goals, keep in mind the acronym SMART. Goals should be

>> **Specific:** For example, don't simply say, "I want to lose weight." State how much weight you want to lose.

>> **Measurable:** Set a number; when you've reached the number, you know you've reached your goal.

>> **Attainable:** The goal you set should be reachable yet challenging, so that you're likely to achieve it with your efforts.

>> **Realistic:** The goal should be doable. Start with small goals that fit in with your real-life circumstances.

>> **Time-frame specific:** A deadline for your goal can keep you working toward it. Set short-term goals, such as 1 week, so that you see progress.

You may want to choose short-term goals for the day or week and long-term goals for the month or year. For example, if your goal is to lose 10 pounds this year, you'll want to set clear weekly targets to meet that goal in terms of diet and exercise.

Considering Different Types of Exercise

When you've started moving more often in your daily life, you may want to add some more structured exercise. This doesn't have to be a crazy commitment. It could be as simple as following a regular walking plan, taking a water aerobics class, or doing yoga.

In the following sections, we give you an overview of the three basic types of exercise: aerobic, resistance, and flexibility. All three types are important for different reasons.

Aerobic exercise: Getting the blood moving

Aerobic exercise gets your heart pounding and your large muscles moving. It includes walking, running, swimming, bicycling, skiing, and many other activities.

Why is aerobic exercise so awesome? It's the double-whammy effect. It increases your muscles' ability take up glucose from your blood. It also makes the cells in your muscles and liver more sensitive to insulin. So, your blood glucose is lower and you don't need as much insulin.

Aerobic exercise is also the best way to burn calories to lose or maintain weight. It can also benefit your immune system and lungs.

REMEMBER

The American Diabetes Association recommends that most people with type 2 diabetes exercise 150 minutes or more a week. The exercise should be moderate to vigorous, and it should be spread out over at least 3 days a week.

Try any or all of these aerobic exercises to get your heart pumping:

>> Take a fast-paced walk outside.

>> Go dancing, or better yet, have a dance party in your living room.

>> Play golf or squash.

>> Swim in your local pool.

>> Ride your bike or jump on a stationary bike at the gym.

>> Grab your kids and play Wii or other exercise video games.

>> Walk with your friend at an indoor mall if the weather stinks.

REMEMBER

You may see the benefits to your blood glucose immediately after working out and for up to a day after. Also, long-term aerobic exercise can improve your A1C, blood lipids, and blood pressure.

Resistance exercise: Building strength

Resistance exercise, sometimes called strength training, includes using free weights, weight machines, and resistance bands. Don't assume you have to own a gym membership to perform resistance exercises, though. Lots of resistance exercises simply use your own body weight to make your muscles work. Examples include arm raises and leg lifts.

Resistance exercises are important for people with diabetes because they're more likely to have low muscle strength and an accelerated decline in muscle strength.

The benefits of resistance training include improvements in building muscles, body composition, strength, physical function, mental health, bone mineral density, insulin sensitivity, blood pressure, blood lipids, and cardiovascular health.

In people with type 2 diabetes, resistance training can improve blood glucose, insulin resistance, fat mass, blood pressure, and lean body mass.

Here are some resistance exercises you can do that don't require any special equipment:

>> Planks to strengthen your core and entire body

>> Squats to work your legs and entire body

>> Leg lifts to target your core and legs

>> Arm raises to strengthen your shoulders and arm muscles

REMEMBER

The American Diabetes Association recommends that most people with type 2 diabetes do resistance exercise at least 2 days, but preferably 3 days, a week. The exercises should be moderate to vigorous in intensity, and you should include eight to ten different exercises on your resistance-training day. Do 10 to 15 repetitions of each exercise for one to three sets.

What's the difference between an exercise, a repetition, and a set?

>> An **exercise** is the movement you're doing, such as a squat or an arm raise.

>> A **repetition** is how many times you do that movement (for example, 10–15 arm raises).

>> A **set** is a group of repetitions. So, 10–15 arm raises would be one set. You may want to do one to three sets of a particular exercise.

TIP

The American Diabetes Association says that doing both aerobic and resistance exercises may offer the most benefit to people with type 2 diabetes. Instead of either/or, try to do both! (See the preceding section for more about aerobic exercises.)

Flexibility and balance exercises: Improving range of motion

Flexibility and balance exercises are activities that stretch your muscles and joints. Examples include yoga, Pilates, and tai chi. Flexibility exercises can also be as simple as stretching your legs, arms, and neck. Balance exercises can be as simple as standing on one leg at a time or walking backward or sideways.

These exercises can be whole-body workouts like tai chi or yoga, but they can also be part of your warm-up or cool-down routine for aerobic or resistance exercises. (Find out more about warm-ups and cool-downs in the following section.)

The benefits of flexibility exercises may be particularly important for older people with type 2 diabetes because they may not have as much elasticity as they once did. Stretching can increase range of motion and the flexibility of joints. That may extend to balance training, which can reduce the rate of falls.

Some studies have shown that yoga may improve blood glucose, blood lipids, and body composition in people with type 2 diabetes.

REMEMBER

The American Diabetes Association recommends that people with diabetes do flexibility and balance exercises at least 2–3 days a week. You can do them as long as you like, and these exercises can be of light to moderate intensity.

TIP

When you're stretching, try to focus on your breath. Slow your breathing and be deliberate about breathing in and breathing out. Stretch to the point of tightness, but never pain, in your muscles and joints.

Completing a Well-Rounded Workout: Warm Up, Work Out, Cool Down

Exercise should happen in stages such as warming up, working out, and cooling down. You don't want to just jog out your front door or jump into an aerobics class cold. Ideally, you can plan a few minutes at the beginning and end of your exercise to help your body regulate and stretch.

The following sections walk you through the three phases you should include in your workout.

Warming up

A warm-up should include 5–10 minutes of stretching and very light aerobic exercise to get your heart pumping. If you have time, you should always warm up before aerobic or resistance exercises.

The goal of warming up is to increase your heart rate, warm up your muscles, and prevent injuries. (Find out more about heart rate in the "Working out" section.) Many people incorporate the stretching and flexibility exercises mentioned in the previous sections.

For example, you could roll your head and neck in a circular motion. Stretch your arms up and out to your side and then meet your hands overhead. Bend over slowly and try to touch your toes (or at least as close as feels comfortable). Walking or jogging in place may get your heart rate up; doing a lower-intensity version of your exercises can do the same.

Working out

Each person's goal for working out may be different based on his or her overall health, fitness, and age. Your goals may change based on time constraints or even your energy level during the day. Ideally, most people with type 2 diabetes should try to hit the American Diabetes Association's target of 150 minutes of exercise a week.

But how do you know how hard or easy to work out? It may help to think of exercise in terms of reaching your target heart rate. Ask your physician what your target heart rate should be during exercise. Then you can measure it during exercise to see whether you're in a good range.

Heart rate devices often come on fitness trackers these days, but you can also measure your heart rate without any fancy devices. (Find out more about fitness trackers in the "Getting detailed feedback from fitness trackers and apps" section later in this chapter.)

Here's how to measure your heart rate:

1. **Put the tips of your first two fingers lightly over a blood vessel in your neck, just to the left or right side. Or put your two fingers on the pulse spot on your wrist below your thumb.**

2. **Count how many beats you feel over 10 seconds.**

3. **Multiply by 6.**

   Now you know your beats per minute, which is your heart rate.

Your heart rate during exercise should be higher than your resting heart rate. Ask your physician or diabetes educator to determine the best number to shoot for while exercising. This can tell you when to slow down or push yourself harder during physical activity.

TIP

Another way to make sure you're not exerting yourself too hard is to do the talk test: You should be able to talk while exercising.

Cooling down

During cool-down, you want to lower your heart rate and slow down your breathing. To do this, you may want to exercise at a lower intensity for a few minutes. For example, if you're running, cool down by lightly jogging. If you're briskly walking, cool down by slowing walking.

TIP

Incorporate stretches during cool-down to avoid injuries and lengthen muscles. The same exercises you did during warm-up may work perfectly for cool-down, too.

Motivators to Keep You Going

Keeping up with regular exercise can be one of the hardest things to do. Why? One of the reasons may be that we lack motivation over time. Sometimes we may feel too out of shape or overweight to even begin. Sometimes we may get discouraged because we don't see the results we want right away. Or sometimes, everyday logistics and life pressures get in the way of our best intentions.

To stay motivated, it helps to have realistic goals. (Read about the benefits of setting goals and how to set them in the "Thinking about your fitness goals" section earlier in this chapter.) These goals can be based on targets you want to achieve in your diabetes care, your overall health, or just how you look and feel.

REMEMBER

You want your goals to be specific, measurable, and attainable. You may also want to set short-term goals to keep you on track each week.

Envisioning the health benefits

Some of the best motivators for exercising are the clear benefits to your blood glucose and other health measures. Exercise is so good for people with type 2 diabetes in terms of their A1C, blood pressure, blood lipids, and risk factors for cardiovascular disease. That's why the American Diabetes Association recommends that you do it 150 minutes a week!

Some people find their motivation in thinking about how staying healthy may help them enjoy their family and friends into old age. They want to improve their health so they can take their kids fishing, be there for their kids' weddings, or hold their grandchildren. Being around for these times, whether they're run-of-the-mill activities or special events, can be the encouragement you need to exercise and take care of your health in other ways. Use whatever positive outcomes you need to in order to get and stay motivated.

Getting help from a professional

TIP

If you're new to exercise, you may benefit from seeing a fitness professional — anyone from an exercise physiologist to a personal trainer who works at your local YMCA.

An exercise physiologist is a health professional with a bachelor's or master's degree who has received certification in exercise physiology. Read more about exercise physiologists and their part on your healthcare team in Chapter 3.

A personal trainer helps motivate, develop, and safely follow an exercise routine. Personal trainers can come to your home or work at gyms. You may also find specific instructors, like a yoga teacher or water aerobics teacher, helpful in setting goals or making fitness recommendations.

Any fitness professional should begin her work with you by evaluating your fitness and health. She can help you set realistic goals, develop a tailor-made program, and offer motivation for sticking to your routine. Don't be shy about asking whether the trainer has experience helping people with type 2 diabetes.

Boosting your mood

Exercise improves your outlook and combats symptoms of depression. When you exercise, you may feel better because you're distracted from stresses and feel empowered about yourself and your activity. Your brain and hormones change, too, releasing feel-good hormones called *endorphins*.

Some studies show that exercising outside or in nature really helps with mood and energy. But to be honest, any type of exercise helps you feel better.

In one study, overweight people with type 2 diabetes who tried to lose more than 7 percent of their body weight and exercised more than 175 minutes a week reported improvements in quality of life and symptoms of depression.

Getting support from friends and family

Support from friends and family can help you achieve your fitness goals. You may think you can go it alone, but outside encouragement and a sense of community and responsibility can help.

There is not a one-size-fits-all prescription for support. Support could mean the inspiration you find from walking with a co-worker during lunch. Support could mean the sense of purpose you find from an online community of people with type 2 diabetes who are trying to lose weight or get in shape. Support could mean the camaraderie you feel from joining a YMCA where you try new classes or just cycle on a stationary bike next to someone else. Support could also mean having a fitness partner who is relying on you to show up. For example, if someone is expecting you to do a yoga class on Saturday morning or walk at lunch, you may feel more accountable and, therefore, more likely to follow through with exercise plans.

TIP

You may need to look outside your immediate support network of friends and family — and that can be challenging because living with type 2 diabetes is new and unpredictable. Don't get discouraged. You're on the right path if you're taking steps to get moving.

Getting detailed feedback from fitness trackers and apps

Personal fitness trackers (also called activity monitors) that you wear on your wrist or waistband can help you stay motivated. They measure your daily activity and workout in steps, distance, calories burned, and the minutes that you were actively moving throughout the day.

Just by wearing a fitness tracker, you can get a snapshot of your fitness throughout the day. People also like fitness trackers because they measure activity and help you determine whether you've met certain goals. For example, you may have a goal of reaching 10,000 steps a day or exercising for 30 minutes. A fitness tracker can help you determine whether you achieved your goal.

A fitness tracker can also help you connect the dots between your activity and your health goals, including your diabetes. For example, you may feel amazing when you've worked out for 45 minutes. Comparing that activity to your blood glucose tests can help you see that your blood glucose is lower when you exercise.

Most fitness trackers come with an app that you download on your phone to see more details about your activity.

Here are some special features of fitness trackers to consider if you decide to invest in one:

>> A heart rate monitor built into the device can be helpful.

>> Sleep trackers measure how much you sleep during the night.

>> Several models allow you to log your food and meals on the app.

>> Ways to stay connected with friends are also popular. Some models let you connect with others, message to offer support, and compare workouts.

>> Looks matter because you'll be wearing your tracker all day (and sometimes all night). Choose a style that speaks to you!

TIP

You may not need a fancy model or even a fitness tracker at all. Apple and Google both have apps that allow you to track your movements based just on carrying your phone with you throughout the day.

You can find other fitness apps, separate from fitness trackers, that can help you measure and meet your fitness goals. Check out iTunes or Google Play for ones that are highly rated and popular.

5

Finding Support

Manage your emotions, handle stress, avoid diabetes burnout, reach out to others with diabetes, and practice self-compassion.

Develop skills to become a more supportive caretaker or spouse of someone with diabetes.

Discover how type 2 diabetes is different in children and teens and find out how the whole family can offer support.

Find out why some common misconceptions about diabetes are incorrect.

Chapter **14**

Managing Your Emotions and Mental Health

How did you feel when you were first diagnosed with type 2 diabetes? Likely, the diagnosis elicited strong emotions and concerns. Perhaps you felt like it wasn't fair or wasn't real. Perhaps you felt lonely or overwhelmed.

Everyone feels differently when they're diagnosed with diabetes, in part because the circumstances of diagnosis can vary widely. Some people may find out they have diabetes because they notice complications such as changes in their vision or high blood pressure. Other people may find out they have diabetes because they check into the hospital or see their doctor for another concern. Some individuals may realize that they've been at risk for diabetes for years because they have a family history of diabetes or because they're older.

Whatever the circumstances, it's shocking to find out that you have a chronic condition. It's a burden to discover that you need to take care of your body and mind in new ways to stay healthy. And people feel varying degrees of anger, denial, fear, and stress about diabetes.

Recognizing these emotions can help you channel this energy in positive ways. You may feel like your diagnosis is a sudden wake-up call to take better care of yourself, or it may take a while to figure out your strategy.

Your emotional well-being is integral to your health. When you feel good, you're more likely to take better care of your blood glucose and other areas of diabetes management. When you let stress, depression, denial, or other negative emotions get the best of you, your health suffers, and you're more likely to struggle with controlling your diabetes.

In this chapter, you discover emotions common to people with diabetes — as well as strategies for coping with them. Stress, anger, denial, and even diabetes burnout are part of the discussion, as well as more serious concerns such as depression and anxiety disorders.

Support groups for people with type 2 diabetes abound, in communities and online. In this chapter, you find out about how reaching out to others can help. Finally, we explain the importance of being kind to yourself — it can't be overemphasized.

Getting in Touch with How You Feel

Ask yourself how *you* feel about your diabetes. What does that mean? Well, certain emotions probably pop into your heart and mind when you think about your diabetes. What are they, and how do they make you feel?

Think about common stressors, those moments in the day when you get frustrated. Some of these circumstances may be out of your control, but naming them is a first step in getting in touch with your emotions. Alternatively, identify those times when you feel satisfied and unconcerned about your health.

You may want to change your attitude and behaviors, or you may be doing a great job managing certain circumstances, and you want to do more of that positive coping.

Getting in touch with how you feel may seem like a luxury, but it's a practical step in better managing your health. Use the following questions to help you get in touch with your feelings:

>> How do you feel when you think about your diabetes and your future?

>> What parts of your care make you the most stressed and concerned?

>> What parts of your care make you feel most empowered?

>> Are you dealing with common everyday stressors? If you could, how would you change these stressors?

>> If you could pick one thing to improve, what would it be?

Facing Feelings of Anger and Denial

Anger and denial are common feelings when people are first diagnosed with diabetes, but these feelings can occur throughout a lifetime of living with a chronic condition.

If you consistently experience feelings of denial or anger, talk to your healthcare provider about coping strategies. Join a support group of other people with diabetes, online or in your neighborhood, so you can express your feelings with people who may be experiencing the same things.

Acknowledging feelings of anger

Anger is that genuine feeling of infuriation and annoyance about diabetes. You may feel anger at your physician or diabetes educator for delivering an unwanted diagnosis or bad news about a complication. You may feel angry about your health insurance if you don't have enough coverage for diabetes supplies and treatment. You may feel angry with your family, friends, and co-workers if they're unsympathetic and unsupportive of your efforts to eat healthy and exercise.

You'll definitely feel angry with yourself. Feeling angry about your diabetes is normal because you can't always control it. Despite your best efforts to lower your blood glucose, eat healthy foods, and exercise, you'll have days when your numbers are off. It's frustrating, but it happens to everyone.

Anger can be positive if it inspires you to change your behavior or environment, but it can be negative if it overwhelms you and paralyzes you in a state of hostility. Recognize that anger is common and find new ways to channel that powerful energy.

Here are some tips for alleviating anger:

>> Try to recognize common triggers by writing down episodes or circumstances when you become angry. Is there a pattern?

>> Try to avoid blurting out criticisms and frustrations in the heat of the moment. Take deep breaths and collect your thoughts before following the next two steps.

>> If another person says or does things to make you angry, try to talk with them about it in a calm moment. Try not to place blame, and be specific and kind.

>> Take a timeout or count to 10. (Get more strategies for de-stressing in the "Managing Stress" section later in this chapter.)

>> Focus on actions and solutions to avoid or lessen anger in stressful moments.

Dealing with feelings of denial

Denial is another emotion that people with type 2 diabetes commonly experience as they begin to cope with diabetes. You have so much new information to absorb — and the education itself can be overwhelming. You may also feel scared about the path forward, including the risk of complications.

Although denial is a natural emotion when you're given shocking or unwanted news, it's not a healthy long-term strategy. Denying you have diabetes won't help you take care of your blood glucose and avoid complications. Denial only gets in your way. After all, diabetes is largely a self-care condition. You are the primary caretaker of your body.

Denial can take many forms. Perhaps you've tried to wish away your diabetes or just not think about it. Or perhaps you've told yourself and others that you'll take care of your diabetes later. This is particularly dangerous because the symptoms of diabetes can go unnoticed while still causing long-term complications or deterioration of blood vessels. Still others may feel that they've had an incorrect diagnosis or their providers don't know what they're talking about. These are all typical feelings of denial that many people with diabetes experience.

You can move past denial by revisiting your diabetes care plan. Remind yourself of your blood glucose goals, such as an A1C below 7. Try to focus on why that number is important — such as preventing complications like eye or kidney disease. Strategize for ways that you'll reach that goal, such as exercising a little bit each day or eating smaller portions or taking your medications on schedule.

Tell others, such as your healthcare provider and friends or family, that you're struggling with feelings of denial. Enlist the help of a certified diabetes educator (CDE) to refresh your diabetes care plan — and brainstorm on ways to meet your daily goals.

Managing Stress

Stress is an all too common emotion in our lives. Everyone deals with the stresses of work, family, friends, and other commitments. However, people with diabetes may be more affected by stress because it impacts both body and mind.

In the body, stress causes the release of hormones that can raise blood glucose. In addition, stress can make it more difficult to effectively manage a chronic condition such as diabetes in which you need to eat healthy foods, exercise, and sleep well. Even though you know you should maintain your healthy habits, stress can undermine your good intentions and management plans — and result in higher blood glucose.

Stress is individual. We all perceive different situations as stressful and have different responses to stress. Something that may be inherently stressful to you, like going to the doctor, may be reassuring and comforting to another person. It all depends on your environment and mood. Also, something that stresses you out today could feel totally fine tomorrow.

Believe it or not, you already have a toolbox of strategies for managing stress. We all have strategies from our upbringing, values, and life experiences. Some of these strategies may be proven winners for managing stress, like laughing out loud, praying, or meditating, while others, like drinking too much or smoking, may create other stressors.

Luckily, several useful tools can help you manage stress in the short and long term. Here are a few you may find helpful:

>> Laugh. Smile. Share a joke or anecdote about your day with a friend or look for the humor in situations.

>> Talk to someone — a spouse, a sibling, a support group, or others — about your stress and feelings.

>> Be mindful and live in the moment. (Read more about mindfulness in the section "Being Kind to Yourself" later in the chapter.)

>> Communicate with others in positive, respectful ways.

>> Get some exercise (see the following section).

>> Take time to relax by scheduling "me" time (reading a good book, soaking in a bubble bath) or time with others (girls' night out or a walk with friends).

>> Slow down your breathing and deeply breathe in and out for several minutes.

>> Practice progressive muscle relaxation in which you close your eyes while focusing on certain areas of your body such as your mouth, shoulders, and feet. Inhale and tense the muscles in those areas; then release those muscles as you exhale.

>> Meditate, pray, or find other ways to refocus inward on positive thoughts and actions.

Choosing alcohol or tobacco to relieve stress is unhealthy for people with diabetes. Drinking in moderation is fine (no more than one drink for adult women per day and no more than two drinks per day for adult men). However, drinking alcohol can increase your risk for lows and highs and weight gain. Lowered inhibitions while drinking excessively could also derail your efforts to eat healthy and exercise. Tobacco increases your risk of cardiovascular disease and early death.

REMEMBER

Throughout the book, we tell you to exercise. Not only does exercise help you physically — by losing weight and maintaining a healthy blood glucose level — but it also helps you mentally — by boosting your mood and lowering your stress. When you exercise, your brain produces chemicals called *endorphins*, which make you feel good.

Exercise can help you combat stress by focusing your mind on something other than the stress at hand. You may feel more calm and meditative, or you may feel energized. Either way, you're less likely to think about your daily irritations and struggles. Exercise can also help you sleep better, which can help you feel less stressed throughout the day.

Recognizing Diabetes Distress and Burnout

Diabetes distress, also called *diabetes burnout*, is a term for the feelings of frustration, worry, and fear that come with managing a chronic condition such as diabetes. These feelings are common; 18–45 percent of people with diabetes report experiencing diabetes distress.

Diabetes distress is a distinct set of emotions that is unique to people with type 1 and type 2 diabetes. The unpredictability of blood glucose levels and the stresses of everyday life can wear on people with diabetes. They can lead to a feeling of burnout where you feel overwhelmed and fed up, which sometimes stops people from taking care of themselves. This in turn can lead to higher A1C and other complications.

It's normal to feel overwhelmed by the responsibility and duty of taking care of yourself 24/7. Watching what you eat, trying to exercise more, and checking blood glucose can feel like too much work.

It's also normal to feel frustrated by the way your friends, family, or complete strangers may treat you differently because of your diabetes. Someone may tell you that you shouldn't eat a certain food or shame you about your behavior. That's not fair or kind.

It's also normal to feel fearful of the complications of diabetes, such as heart or kidney disease. You may worry that you'll have an episode of low blood glucose and not be able to treat it adequately.

Although diabetes distress is common, you still need to address it. You'll want to recognize and cope with diabetes distress so that it doesn't get in the way of your diabetes self-care. For example, high levels of diabetes distress may prevent people from taking their medications as directed and are linked to higher A1C and poorer exercise and eating habits.

Tell your provider if you're experiencing symptoms of diabetes distress. A questionnaire called the Diabetes Distress Scale (DDS) may help measure your feeling of distress and clarify areas that cause you the most hardship. Your healthcare provider may use it, but you can also access it online at the Behavioral Diabetes Institute (www.behavioraldiabetes.org).

Ask for a referral to a diabetes educator, who can identify areas of stress and propose solutions to alleviate diabetes distress. If working with a diabetes educator isn't helpful, you may ask to see a mental health specialist. Diabetes distress is nothing to be ashamed of, and you shouldn't be embarrassed to talk about it with members of your healthcare team — or friends and family.

TIP

Talk to your diabetes educator or other healthcare provider if you're experiencing diabetes distress. Measuring your diabetes distress and finding ways to alleviate these emotions can help.

WARNING

Don't assume your physician will ask you about diabetes distress. In one study, 45 percent of patients reported diabetes distress and yet only 24 percent said their healthcare teams asked them about it.

Looking at Depression and Anxiety Disorders

Anger, denial, stress, and diabetes burnout (all of which are addressed earlier in the chapter) aren't the only emotions people with diabetes experience. Separate from those emotions are the clinical disorders depression and anxiety.

People with diabetes are twice as likely to experience depression as people without diabetes. Anxiety symptoms and disorders are also common in people with diabetes. No one knows exactly why depression and anxiety commonly coexist with diabetes. The causes of these mental health disorders are also unknown, although contributors include certain medications, family history, and living with a chronic disease.

Knowing the symptoms of depression

Depression can happen at any time, either immediately after your diagnosis or after you've been living with diabetes for many years. Not everyone experiences depression in the same way or for the same amount of time. However, there are common symptoms of depression:

» You don't enjoy things that normally make you happy.

» You're tired during the day, and you have trouble falling asleep or you sleep all the time.

» You don't enjoy eating foods that you once adored, and you eat much more or less than usual.

» You may lose or gain a significant amount of weight.

» You have difficulty concentrating, sitting still, or making seemingly straightforward decisions.

» You don't feel good about yourself, and you may even feel like everyone else would be better off without you.

» You think about harming yourself or feel suicidal.

Depression is one of the most common mental health disorders in the United States, affecting at least 16 million adults each year. It is also treatable, so talk to your healthcare provider if you have any of these symptoms. You find out more about treatments later in this chapter.

TECHNICAL
STUFF

Depression and diabetes are *bi-directional*. People with diabetes are more likely to have depression. But people with depression, a history of depression, or who take antidepressant medications are also more likely to have type 2 diabetes. It goes both ways.

Introduction to anxiety disorders

Anxiety disorders are the most common mental health illnesses in the United States, affecting at least 18 million adults each year. They include general anxiety disorder, obsessive-compulsive disorder, and many others.

Some are specific to diabetes such as an obsession with checking your blood glucose numbers, keeping them on target, or having a fear of insulin injections. One study found that 19 percent of people with type 1 or type 2 diabetes had generalized anxiety disorder during their lifetimes.

If your worries, anxieties, and fears get in the way of your life, talk to your physician. He may be able to help, or he may refer you to a mental health professional.

Treating depression and other mental health disorders

Talk to your primary care provider about symptoms of depression or anxiety disorders. It may seem challenging or intimidating to carve out time during your regular checkup, but it's important to discuss your concerns. Your mental state and your emotions have an effect on your physical health, including your blood glucose levels.

Your primary care provider may feel comfortable diagnosing and prescribing a medication. Or she may refer you to a mental health professional such as a psychiatrist, psychologist, licensed social worker, or therapist.

Talking through your emotions and feelings with a professional can help treat mental disorders. *Cognitive behavioral therapy* is a common technique in which you modify your thoughts and change your behaviors. It has been shown to ease the symptoms of depression in people with various disorders, including diabetes. One study showed it has positive effects on anxiety, well-being, and diabetes distress in people with type 1 or type 2 diabetes.

Medications such as antidepressants can help rebalance chemicals in the brain and body. Many people find that a combination of talk therapy and medication helps.

Reaching Out to Others

Talking and sharing experiences with others is one of the most common ways of coping with type 2 diabetes. Many people feel like they're alone with their diagnosis or diabetes care until they make connections with others. You can connect with others through support groups that meet in person or online.

Joining a local support group

In this day and age of digital friendships and virtual connections, you may appreciate the chance to connect in person with other people who have diabetes. If nothing else, you can exchange a sympathetic smile with someone else who's dealing with a situation similar to yours, or you can receive a hug from an understanding group leader.

TIP

Ask your primary care provider or diabetes educator for names of support groups in your area. Hospitals are also good sources for this information.

A diabetes education class may be the first place that you meet others with type 2 diabetes in your community. The class instructor should offer suggestions for finding local support groups, but you should also feel free to ask. Don't be shy about turning to the people next to you to see whether they might be interested in joining you or helping you find a local group.

The American Diabetes Association hosts hundreds of events throughout the year where the organization raises money and awareness for diabetes. The events are a great opportunity to meet others with type 2 diabetes by participating or volunteering your time. There are Diabetes Expos where you can find out about the latest information on diabetes, camps for kids, and bicycle tours and walks for all ages. Check them out at www.diabetes.org.

Connecting with others in online support groups

Going online is a wonderful way to find others with type 2 diabetes going through the same emotions and experiences. You'll find discussions about food, exercise, blood glucose numbers, and more. The advantages of these online support groups are that you can be anonymous and you have access 24/7.

TIP

You can find support groups on the American Diabetes Association's website at http://community.diabetes.org.

Being Kind to Yourself

Thinking positively and taking positive actions are important for your diabetes. Don't underestimate the power of being kind and compassionate to yourself. After all, *you* are the most important part of your diabetes care. If you feel good about yourself, you're more likely to take care of your blood glucose and make other healthy choices.

In the following sections, we give you some tips for taking care of yourself, in the big picture and in smaller moments of stress and uncertainty. (Check out Chapters 15 and 19 for advice on dealing with family members and co-workers, respectively.)

Gaining education and empowerment

Educating yourself about diabetes is an important step in taking care of your health. Just reading this book is a step forward in learning more about how to eat healthy foods, exercise more, and check your blood glucose.

TIP

Take a diabetes education class so you can find out more about type 2 diabetes. Ask your CDE whether she can recommend new tips or techniques for taking care of your diabetes or managing complications. Subscribe to a magazine like the American Diabetes Association's *Diabetes Forecast* (www.diabetesforecast.org) so you can receive healthy living tips in your mailbox every other month.

REMEMBER

The more you educate yourself about diabetes, the more empowered you may feel to make changes and take healthy steps. Education is the key to feeling empowered in managing your diabetes on a day-to-day basis, from keeping track of your blood glucose levels to building a healthcare team you trust.

Taking time for yourself

With the daily demands of taking care of your diabetes, you may find that it's harder to make time for yourself. However, it's just as important to carve time out of the day to relax, rejuvenate, and refresh. It may help with your stress levels and diabetes distress as well.

Taking "me" time means taking a break from work or caring for others like children or spouses. It's an escape from the daily demands of work and life. Some people like to take a walk, read a book, draw a bath, or just sit quietly. Others find that meditation and listening to music are good ways to spend "me" time. You may have to schedule "me" time so it actually happens in your busy day. It could be 5 minutes or 30 minutes, once a week or even every day.

Trying mindfulness and meditation

Mindfulness is the act of being present in the moment, focusing on what you're doing and noting each particular detail. You pay attention to your thoughts, as well as what's going on around you. You can be mindful doing anything, whether reading to your kids at night or checking your blood glucose or mowing the lawn.

In the current age of multitasking, mindfulness has garnered attention for helping people live in the present and focus on what's important. It seems like everyone is embracing mindfulness, from schools to workplaces.

Mindfulness may help people with diabetes recognize how their own bodies react to changes in blood glucose, food, or exercise. It may help some people focus positively on eating nutritious, delicious foods or some other aspect of diabetes self-management. In a small study in New Zealand, people with type 2 diabetes who practiced mindful self-compassion had improvements in depression, distress, and A1C.

Meditation is another practice that can help relieve stress and create a sense of empowerment. During meditation, you focus your mind. You may try to relax your body and use your breath to focus inward and release other thoughts. People also use meditation to improve their health, from lowering blood pressure to reducing pain. People with diabetes may find meditation helpful for all these reasons and more, including a sense of physical and mental calmness.

Chapter **15**

Getting Support, Giving Support

iabetes touches almost everyone in the United States today. You'd be hard-pressed to find someone who doesn't have a relative, neighbor, or friend with type 2 diabetes. You may have diabetes yourself, or you may be caring for someone with diabetes. Either way, diabetes affects all of us in profound ways, especially families.

Diabetes is a family disease for several reasons. Type 2 diabetes runs in families, so you're more likely to have diabetes if your mother, father, or sibling has it. Obesity also runs in families, so you're more likely to be overweight if you have a sibling or parent with extra pounds. Having an overweight spouse may also increase your chances of being overweight. You're more likely to develop type 2 diabetes if you're overweight or obese.

As important as the genetic factors are, the entire family feels it when just one person has diabetes. Diabetes doesn't happen in a bubble — and you can't take a pill to cure it. Instead, you must make daily changes to your lifestyle and health to manage type 2 diabetes. Family members, including spouses, are keenly aware of the changes that come with type 2 diabetes, whether they're fluctuations in mood, new medication routines, or stresses associated with food and exercise.

Learning to communicate effectively as someone with diabetes or as a spouse or relative of someone with diabetes is important. In this chapter, we provide tips for educating your family about your diabetes. Caregivers and spouses, there's a section for you, too. You find out the best ways to offer support and encouragement to your loved one with diabetes. We specifically discuss helping children and teens manage their type 2 diabetes in the next chapter.

Turning to Your Family for Support

Your family can be a fantastic source of support, or it can feel like they're bringing you down. More likely, it's something in between. We love our families, but they can be frustrating sometimes, too!

Realizing that you'll need to take your family into account when you have diabetes may be one of the first steps in seeking support. Other key elements include: education, communication, and eating healthy foods and exercising together.

Telling your friends and family about your diagnosis

There isn't a rule for which people to tell about your diabetes, although most people would agree that telling your spouse or partner is important. You might also consider telling people with whom you live closely such as roommates or your best friend. A good rule of thumb may be to tell people who can offer support and help you navigate diabetes. More support can help you manage your diabetes, and cope with the inevitable frustrations and problems that can come up.

You can be fairly straightforward in your description when talking to a friend or loved one: "I found out that I have type 2 diabetes, and I'm taking steps to manage my blood glucose by eating healthy, exercising more, and taking medications." Be prepared for questions — or silence. Some people may have tons of questions about diabetes and how it impacts you. Other people may not know what to say in that moment. Feel free to tell that person that you're learning about diabetes as you go, too.

Educating your family

Your family may need to learn about diabetes just as you had to learn about diabetes when you were diagnosed. They may not know anything about the cause, diagnosis, management, or treatment of diabetes. Or they may have preconceptions about diabetes that aren't accurate or fair. They may be scared about complications, just as you may be.

TIP

Educating your family about diabetes is a way to open up a conversation. Each member of your family should understand what diabetes is, how it's managed, and how to handle emergencies.

Feel free to tell them about diabetes in your own words or encourage them to seek out their own resources. Websites that educate about the basics of diabetes such as the American Diabetes Association's website (www.diabetes.org) are great places to start. Books like this one or magazines such as *Diabetes Forecast* are other good tools. Online message boards are another source of education and support.

If you feel comfortable, ask a family member such as a spouse or sibling to go with you to your next healthcare appointment. Together or separately, keep a running tally of questions or concerns to bring with you when you visit your physician.

Consider bringing a family member to a diabetes education class so he or she can hear about the basics of diabetes and the steps you'll be taking to manage diabetes through healthy eating, exercise, medications, and checking your blood glucose. Many diabetes education classes encourage family members to attend.

REMEMBER

Emergencies are another topic that you'll want to talk about with your family. Tell your family members about hypoglycemia — as well as its warning signs. (See Chapter 8 for details about hypoglycemia.) Sometimes you may not realize that you're having a low blood glucose level, but your family members may pick up on mood changes and/or fatigue, which can signal a low. Make sure they know what to do if you're having a low, such as making sure you get an appropriate snack or glucose gel.

Opening the lines of communication

An open flow of communication is important for all families, but particularly for ones navigating diabetes. Recognize that mood changes and stress are common symptoms of managing a chronic condition such as diabetes. Talking about your feelings may help you, as well as the people closest to you, feel better.

You may occasionally feel grumpy because of your diabetes or because of all the things you have to deal with on top of your diabetes. These feelings are normal, so try to give yourself a break, and ask your loved ones for extra empathy on those days.

Some family members may show their concern by frequently asking you about your diabetes or reminding you to do certain things. Some people may go so far as to tell you what you should and shouldn't do. These folks are sometimes referred to as the "diabetes police."

If you feel like your family members are being pesky, gently tell them how you feel. Choose a less-heated moment or a time when you and the other person are both relaxed to bring up the topic. Tell them you understand that they're concerned about your health and behaviors; however, you feel like the frequency or tone of their comments and suggestions aren't helpful.

Making healthy food choices together

Choosing healthy foods can be a family affair. After all, everyone needs to eat more wholesome, nutritious foods. You may want to explain to your family that there isn't a special diet that people with diabetes must follow. Instead, people with diabetes should choose healthy foods that are good choices for anyone.

Keep in mind that making food changes can be challenging for individuals — and families. Your family or spouse may be resistant to change if you've been eating a certain way for years (or even a lifetime).

Explain to your family why you're making the changes and ask for their support. If you're the person in charge of meal planning for the family, tell them about the changes you want to make, such as eating more vegetables and whole grains. Ask for their input about what kinds of healthy foods they enjoy and include these foods in new recipes. No one wants to feel like they're being forced to eat certain foods, so giving your family options could alleviate friction.

You may be frustrated when you have to eat smaller portions or cut out certain foods that your spouse or family members enjoy. It can be a real source of tension! Talk to them about these frustrations and ask whether they can be accommodating. It may mean asking them to enjoy less-healthy foods at other times rather than during family meals.

Eating differently may be one of the hardest parts of managing your diabetes, so explain this to your family and ask for their support. Know that eating healthy is good for you and sets an excellent example for your children, spouse, and others. (See more about healthy eating in Chapters 11 and 12.)

Cookbooks such as *Diabetes & Heart Healthy Meals for Two* by the American Diabetes Association and American Heart Association offer recipes that you and your loved one can enjoy together. Other cookbooks that specifically address occasions such as family gatherings and holidays may also offer new recipes. And a meal-planning guide or cookbook such as *The Six O'Clock Scramble Meal Planner* or *Quick Diabetic Recipes For Dummies* (Wiley) can help mothers and fathers cook healthy meals for the whole family.

Exercising together

Exercising is a good way to get your family onboard with your diabetes plan. Just like healthy eating, exercise is good for everyone. And it's one of those things that you can't enjoy too much.

Ask a family member, such as your spouse or significant other or teenage son or daughter, whether he or she would like to join you in exercise. Sometimes an invitation is the best starting point: "Do you want to take a walk with me?" Don't take offense if someone says no. Leave the door open for future participation. However, if someone says yes, then you're off and running (or walking). Having a buddy can be tremendously helpful when starting a new exercise regimen. (See more about exercise in Chapter 13. Also consider picking up a copy of *Diabetes and Keeping Fit For Dummies* [Wiley] for workout routines and fun activities to help you get and stay in shape.)

Planning family activities that involve physical activity will also boost your own fitness. A bike ride, hike, or just hitting a round of putt-putt can be fun adventures for everyone. Turn off the TV and have a dance party or head outside and garden together.

Tips for Caregivers and Spouses

Spouses and caregivers have the unique role of supporting someone with diabetes. The key is, in fact, support. You want to be as supportive as you possibly can for your loved one. Sometimes the way to be supportive may not always be clear, but we give you some tips for navigating this road in the following sections.

Educating yourself

Education is integral to offering meaningful support. You have to understand what you're dealing with before you can jump in and offer your assistance.

Find resources for learning about diabetes by looking online at www.diabetes.org or other websites. Check out books from the library or order a subscription to magazines such as *Diabetes Forecast* (www.diabetesforecast.org) for you and your loved ones. Find recipes online or read cookbooks about diabetes that will help you plan healthy meals for you and your loved ones.

Ask whether you can attend a diabetes education class with your loved one. Seek out community resources such as local health fairs or the American Diabetes Association's Diabetes Expo where you can learn about diabetes from experts.

Be patient with yourself and recognize that you'll experience a learning curve. The education may seem overwhelming at first, but allow yourself time to learn and to breathe. Your spouse or loved one may be experiencing the same feelings.

REMEMBER

People with diabetes can have health issues related to sex such as erectile dysfunction; difficulty with arousal; or pain during intercourse (see Chapters 9 and 10 for more details). If you're a partner of someone with diabetes, these issues can certainly affect you, too. Educate yourself about common sexual health issues and be open to discussing them if they come up. Your partner (or you) may find these topics difficult to discuss, but talking about them is the first step. Effective treatments are available, so encourage your partner to bring up any concerns with his or her physician.

Trying not to be pesky

WARNING

One of the most common traps that spouses and caregivers fall into is becoming the "diabetes police." This term refers to individuals who try to monitor and dictate another person's management of diabetes. Of course, the intent is good: You want to help your spouse or loved one make healthy choices about eating, exercising, or checking blood glucose. However, these suggestions can come across as nagging if they're delivered too frequently or with a harsh tone.

Sometimes a spouse or family member of a person with diabetes will want to call healthcare professionals to offer information about the patient and request feedback. Generally, unless it's an emergency call or the healthcare provider was given explicit permission to do so, he or she may not feel comfortable discussing the patient's health without that person being present. However, the healthcare provider may be open to scheduling a conversation with both the patient and the family member(s). Always check with your loved one first before calling his or her healthcare providers.

TIP

As an alternative, ask your spouse or loved one for concrete examples of how you can be helpful. Start by asking, "What can I do to help you the most in managing your diabetes?" You may be surprised by the answer!

Helping to build a diabetes care team

Ask your loved one or spouse whether he or she would like help building a network of healthcare providers. This can be an overwhelming task in managing diabetes. Finding the right endocrinologist, podiatrist, dentist, or certified diabetes educator (CDE) isn't always easy. An extra set of hands to schedule appointments and find specialists may be welcome.

You may want to ask whether you can attend appointments with your spouse or loved one. Sometimes it can be helpful to have someone else listening to a physician's recommendations or asking pertinent questions. Write down your own concerns beforehand or work on a list of questions with your loved one so you remember your concerns and have time to address them during the appointment.

Seeking out your own support

As caregivers, spouses, and family members, we feel the stress of living with diabetes, too. It's natural to feel overwhelmed by the daily demands of caring for someone else or the pressure and fatigue of worrying about your spouse's health.

TIP

Seek out your own support group in your community or online. Other caregivers and spouses feel the same way you do, and talking with them may help relieve some of the stress or sadness you're experiencing. Talk to a therapist or family counselor to get a professional's perspective and advice on the demands of caregiving on relationships.

Chapter **16**

Raising Children and Teens with Type 2 Diabetes

Twenty years ago, it was unusual for children to have type 2 diabetes. In fact, type 2 diabetes used to be called "adult-onset diabetes" because it almost always occurred in adults.

Today it's a different story: More children than ever have type 2 diabetes, and it's on the rise. A recent study showed the rate of newly diagnosed cases of type 2 diabetes in youth increased by 4.8 percent each year from 2002–2012.

WARNING

According to a 2014 Centers for Disease Control and Prevention (CDC) report card, 5,000 children will be newly diagnosed with type 2 diabetes each year in the United States.

If you're reading this chapter, you may be a parent of a child or teen with type 2 diabetes. In this chapter, we explain how and why type 2 diabetes is different in children; how to take care of your child with type 2 diabetes; and what specific challenges these children and their families face.

Seeing How Type 2 Diabetes Is Different in Children and Teens

Type 2 diabetes is different in children and teens for several reasons, including its progression and its prevalence in certain ethnic minorities. We discuss both aspects later in this section, but first, here are the risk factors for type 2 diabetes in youth:

>> **Ethnicity:** Native American, African American, Asian, and Hispanic youth all have a higher risk for type 2 diabetes than non-Hispanic white youth.

>> **Obesity:** Being overweight as a child increases a person's risk for type 2 diabetes.

>> **Gender:** Girls are more likely to have type 2 diabetes than boys.

>> **Family history:** Kids with parents, siblings, or other family members with type 2 diabetes have a higher risk. If a child's mother had gestational diabetes or type 2 diabetes during pregnancy, the child also has a higher risk.

Studies are showing that type 2 diabetes in children is more aggressive than in adults. It's a double punch. The beta cells that make insulin stop working in children more rapidly than in adults with type 2 diabetes, so it may progress more rapidly or blood glucose may be more difficult to control. Also, youth with type 2 diabetes may develop complications such as eye, heart, and kidney disease sooner than adults with type 2 diabetes throughout the course of their lives.

Many teens diagnosed with type 2 diabetes already have related complications such as high blood pressure, poor blood lipids, and obesity. Therefore, diagnosis and management of type 2 diabetes is critical for helping them lead healthy, productive lives.

In addition to being more aggressive, type 2 diabetes disproportionately affects children of ethnic and racial minorities — and those with lower socioeconomic status.

Despite these risks, children and teens with type 2 diabetes can take steps to manage their blood glucose and reduce the risk of complications. They can change what they eat and how much they exercise. These healthy lifestyle changes should be the focus for teens with diabetes — and their families. Read on for tips about how to address these challenges and help your teen manage her type 2 diabetes.

Helping Your Child or Teen Manage Her Condition

A diagnosis of type 2 diabetes can be shocking for a child — and for his parents and family members. It's unsettling to find out that your child has a chronic condition that needs to be managed on a daily basis. Nevertheless, you can take active steps as a family to help manage blood glucose and reduce the risk of complications.

First steps

Your child may be diagnosed with type 2 diabetes by his pediatrician, during a routine physical school exam, or other circumstance. The American Diabetes Association recommends that children who are 18 and younger and overweight be tested for type 2 diabetes or prediabetes. Your child may be tested because of other risk factors like a family history of type 2 diabetes, race/ethnicity (Native American, African American, Latino, Asian American, Pacific Islander), or a mom who had diabetes during pregnancy.

At the time of diagnosis, your child will receive a full evaluation of any other health risks or complications. This could include a blood sample for lipids, a urine sample for kidney damage, blood pressure measurement, and a dilated eye exam. Your child may see his or her pediatrician for these tests, or he or she may be referred to a pediatric doctor specializing in endocrinology or other areas. For example, your child may need to see a specialist for problems related to the eyes, kidneys, or heart.

Seeing these specialists is part of building a diabetes care team that will probably include a pediatrician or other diabetes care provider, certified diabetes educator (CDE), registered dietitian, and psychologist or social worker.

REMEMBER

The American Diabetes Association recommends an A1C of less than 7.5 percent for children and teens with type 2 diabetes. (For an explanation of A1C, see Chapter 1.)

Focusing on exercise and nutrition

Exercise and nutrition are important for adolescents with type 2 diabetes because they're often overweight, too. The American Academy of Pediatrics (AAP) recommends that children and adolescents with type 2 diabetes exercise (moderately to vigorously) at least 60 minutes a day and limit screen time (non-academic) to less than 3 hours.

Students with type 2 diabetes can play sports and do afterschool activities just like their peers. Talk to your student's coaches or instructors if your child might need care during these activities, based on his or her diabetes medical management plan (see Chapter 16 for more details on these plans).

Just as for adults with diabetes, there is not a specific meal plan for adolescents with type 2 diabetes. Instead, parents should help their child choose wholesome, nutritious foods low in saturated fat and added sugar (see Chapter 12 for more tips on meal planning).

Taking medications

Besides changes to exercise and meals, your adolescent with diabetes may need to take a pill called metformin to treat blood glucose or use insulin injections. Ask your provider if you have any questions about the dose or timing of taking these medications. And see more in Chapter 6 about these specific medications.

Monitoring blood glucose

Whether and how often your child monitors his or her own blood glucose will depend on his or her diabetes management plan and medications. Ask your child's healthcare provider for details. The same guidelines for adults may apply to most youth with type 2 diabetes.

As a parent, you may check your child's blood glucose together (depending on his or her age). Teens may feel comfortable checking and recording their blood glucose on their own. It's a personal decision, so talk with your diabetes care team for guidance, education, and support. Your diabetes educator may be a great source of support for learning how, when, and why to check blood glucose (also see Chapter 7). Also check out more information in Chapter 19 about making a plan for managing type 2 diabetes at school.

TIP

Coming up with a plan for how your child discusses his blood glucose testing ahead of time may relieve some stress. For example, if a friend or stranger asks what he is doing, he might have a straightforward response prepared such as: "I have type 2 diabetes and I check my blood glucose to take care of myself and stay healthy."

Family changes

As a parent, your support and education are critical to helping your adolescent manage his or her diabetes. According to the American Academy of Pediatrics, engaging parents are critical to making needed changes in lifestyle and encouraging children to take their medications as directed.

You, your child, and other family members should try to make lifestyle changes together such as eating healthy foods and exercising regularly. A family-centered approach to nutrition and exercise is essential for children with type 2 diabetes, according to the American Diabetes Association.

REMEMBER

Obesity is one of the leading causes of type 2 diabetes in children, so your child may need to make significant changes in his or her eating habits and physical activity levels to lose weight.

Families can set a good example for children with type 2 diabetes by eating whole-some, nutritious foods in small portions. The same positive eating habits for adults with type 2 diabetes are beneficial for children with type 2 diabetes. Choose low-sodium, low-sugar foods with fewer saturated fats.

Teens have strong opinions, so involve them in decision-making whenever possible. Teach your child how to read food labels: Examine the packages of foods that she enjoys and evaluate those foods' nutrition and calories. Ask your teen to look online for yummy, healthful recipes and cook together when possible. Nutrition starts at home, so try to make renewed efforts to eat healthy foods together as a family.

TIP

It's normal to feel guilt when your child is diagnosed with any chronic disorder, including type 1 or type 2 diabetes. Try to minimize stress and guilt so that you can focus on the important work of helping your child cope with type 2 diabetes. Take care of yourself — emotionally and physically — educate yourself, and consider seeing a mental health specialist for support.

Exercising together can also go a long way toward helping your teen stay more active. Start by asking your teen about her favorite type of exercise, and do that first. On the weekend, plan family adventures that include physical activity such as walks in the park, bike rides, and swimming at the pool in the summer. Turn off the TV and other screens whenever possible and do something active as a family outside.

Education and responsibility

Encourage your child or teen to learn about diabetes by pointing out safe sources of information online. One example is the American Diabetes Association's "Be Healthy Today; Be Healthy For Life" pamphlet at www.diabetes.org. Other online resources include support groups for teens with type 2 diabetes where they can chat about common struggles and questions.

Reinforce the fundamentals of diabetes management for your teen: Eat healthy foods, exercise regularly, remember to take medications, and check your blood glucose.

As your child moves through the teenage years to adulthood, he may struggle with the responsibility of managing a chronic condition such as type 2 diabetes. It's not easy. Be patient and slowly make changes. Point out positive changes and choices so your child feels empowered rather than discouraged. See more about the specific challenges that teens face in the next section.

REMEMBER

You'll want to communicate with your child's teacher, nurse, and other school personnel about her diabetes because she spends the majority of her time at school. Prioritize diabetes management, safety, and academic growth. Check out www.diabetes.org for resources in developing written plans such as a Diabetes Medical Management Plan or Individualized Education Program.

Checkups

Regular checkups are an essential part of your child's type 2 diabetes care. Your child should have a diabetes checkup every 2–3 months, including checks of A1C and blood glucose management, weight, and blood pressure. Your child's physician will probably recommend an annual dilated eye exam, foot exams, and screenings for kidney and cardiovascular disease as appropriate.

Obesity, which is common in children with type 2 diabetes, presents its own health challenges. Overweight children and teens may have sleep apnea, foot problems, and issues with self-esteem or other mental health concerns. Bring up these concerns or problems with your child's physician so he can recommend treatments or specialists.

A recent study found that less than half of children with type 2 diabetes had received an eye exam, even 6 years after diagnosis. Researchers don't know why, but perhaps it's because children (and their parents) must typically take the extra step of seeing a specialist such as an ophthalmologist for this type of dilated eye exam.

REMEMBER

It's important to your child's vision to have regular eye exams. Sometimes eye disease can progress without symptoms, so seeing an eye specialist regularly is critical to maintain vision and treat problems before it's too late.

Acknowledging Challenges that Teens Face

The teenage years are rife with drama, risk taking, and experimentation for any teen. Hormones are in full swing. Teens may feel like their bodies, feelings, and friends change daily. Add a diagnosis of type 2 diabetes to the mix, and your teen may feel completely overwhelmed.

REMEMBER

Hormones change during puberty, affecting all adolescents. The common feelings of moodiness and stress can affect teens with type 2 diabetes, making them feel frustrated about their blood glucose or diabetes, in general. Girls with diabetes may experience changes (up or down) in their blood glucose before and during their menstrual cycles (see more about menstrual cycles in Chapter 9).

Recognizing the challenges that teens typically face can help you communicate and set expectations. Stress, alcohol, tobacco and other drugs, and sexual activity are important topics to discuss with teens with type 2 diabetes.

Stress

Everyone with diabetes experiences stress, and teens are no exception. It's stressful to measure what you eat, how much you exercise, and how much you weigh. These stresses can affect how you feel about yourself — and how you manage your diabetes.

Encourage your teen to combat stress by making healthy choices such as exercising and eating wholesome food. It's not easy to decline a large portion or food high in saturated fats or added sugars when everyone else is eating it. Your child won't always make a perfect decision, so try not to focus on the negative. Focus on and celebrate positive changes such as losing 1 or 2 pounds or lowering A1C.

TIP

Your teen may struggle with telling his friends, and particularly someone he's interested in dating, about diabetes. Diabetes is nothing to be embarrassed about or hide. However, it's a personal decision about who to tell and when to tell them. You may want to practice strategies for telling new people about diabetes with your teen. For example, "I have diabetes, and I manage it by eating well, exercising, and taking medications."

Alcohol and tobacco

It's illegal to sell or serve alcohol to people under 21 years of age in public places, according to state laws. However, some teenagers experiment with alcohol, and they should be aware of the dangers with diabetes.

Alcohol can interfere with diabetes medications, including insulin. It can also make it harder to keep blood glucose in the target range because it can both raise and lower blood glucose to the extremes. Teens with type 2 diabetes need to be aware of the warning signs of very high and very low blood glucose levels and should always be prepared to treat hypoglycemia (see Chapter 8).

Tobacco is also illegal if you're underage, and it can be particularly damaging for teens with type 2 diabetes. Tobacco damages blood vessels and can put increased stress on already weakened blood vessels in people with type 2 diabetes. It's difficult to quit smoking cigarettes or using tobacco, so the best choice is never to start.

TIP

Talk to your teenager about the dangers of alcohol, tobacco, and other drug use. Encourage her to make healthy choices and keep the lines of communication open. Be willing to listen.

Sexual activity

Choosing whether and when to have sex is another decision that your teenager may be faced with. It's an extremely personal decision, but one that hopefully your teenager will feel comfortable discussing with you, a doctor or nurse, or another trusted adult.

Talk to your child about safe sex, which is important for all teens to avoid pregnancy and sexually transmitted diseases like HIV/AIDS. Safe sex is also important for teenage girls with type 2 diabetes to avoid unplanned pregnancies. High blood glucose during pregnancy has risks for the teenage mother, such as high blood pressure and cesarean delivery, and for her baby, such as large birth weight and injuries during birth. Certain medications can also harm the baby during an unplanned pregnancy. (Chapter 9 has more details about diabetes and pregnancy.)

» Seeing the truth about your
  susceptibility to illness

» Remembering that taking insulin
  doesn't equal failure

» Understanding how serious
  diabetes is

Chapter **17**

Debunking Diabetes Myths

Myths and misconceptions about diabetes are everywhere! Myths are problematic because they're widely held beliefs that are actually false. Misconceptions are equally problematic because they're incorrect assumptions based on faulty reasoning or ideas. *False* and *incorrect* are the key points here.

When myths and misconceptions spread about disorders such as diabetes, it's hurtful and unproductive. Perhaps it's because so many people are affected by type 2 diabetes that those falsehoods have such a big impact. Maybe it's because individuals manage their own diabetes, so those incorrect ideas and judgments seem personal. Or perhaps it's because those myths and misconceptions make it appear that having type 2 diabetes is somehow a choice.

In fact, type 2 diabetes is not a choice, according to the American Diabetes Association. The Association and others are committed to dispelling myths and misconceptions about diabetes. You can probably rattle off dozens of misconceptions you've heard in the months or years since your diagnosis. Here, we examine some common diabetes myths and break down why they're wrong, examine the history behind them, and present the facts and latest scientific evidence.

Myth 1: Eating Too Much Sugar Causes Diabetes

Eating too much sugar isn't good for you, but it alone does not cause type 2 diabetes. Let's look at what we know about sugar first. Sugar and starch are the two main types of carbohydrates that our bodies use for energy. Small amounts of sugar are fine, and sugars are found naturally in some foods such as fruit.

Sugar is dangerous because people eat too much of it and because they eat sugar instead of other nutritious foods. In other words, people fill up on sugar and don't have room for the good stuff. Their diets lack wholesome foods that build muscles and bone, promote a healthy immune system, and keep blood vessels clear and free flowing.

Eating too much sugar can also pack on pounds, leading to obesity, which is a risk factor for type 2 diabetes. This is an important piece of the puzzle. However, there are many risk factors for type 2 diabetes beyond obesity and diet.

Native Americans, Asian Americans, African Americans, and Hispanics are more likely to have type 2 diabetes, so your race and ethnicity are important contributors. Your family history — including whether your parents, siblings, aunts, or uncles have type 2 diabetes — is a risk factor, too. Your age is another consideration because your risk for type 2 diabetes increases with age.

Keep in mind that regularly drinking sugary drinks like soda and energy drinks has its own risks. Studies have shown that people who regularly drink sugary drinks, such as one to two cans of soda or more per day, are more likely to develop type 2 diabetes and obesity. Avoid added sugars and, in particular, sugary drinks such as soda to prevent diabetes and better manage your blood glucose and weight if you already have type 2 diabetes.

REMEMBER

Instead of one cause, type 2 diabetes has many risk factors. The more risk factors you have, the more likely you'll have type 2 diabetes someday. However, you can reduce your risk of type 2 diabetes with changes to diet, weight, exercise, and medications.

Myth 2: People with Diabetes Can't Eat Sweets and Chocolate

This could be one of the most frustrating myths about diabetes because it makes people feel bad about their food choices. Here's a scenario that may sound familiar: You've counted your calories for the day, planned ahead to enjoy a special treat, and are just about to take a bite of birthday cake. Then someone turns to you and asks, "Should you be eating that?"

The myth that people with diabetes can't enjoy sweets and chocolate has probably ruined more office parties and birthday celebrations than anyone would care to count. The fact is that eating occasional, small portions of sweets can be part of a healthy diet for anyone, including people with diabetes.

Sweets and chocolates include *added sugar*, which is in many foods besides these treats. Added sugars are in sodas, energy drinks, and iced teas, as well as crackers, bread, granola, and many more products. You can find a line called "Added Sugars" under the "Total Carbohydrate" line on food labels. Try to focus on the grams of added sugar, rather than percent daily value. Keeping added sugars to a minimum is ideal, and the American Heart Association recommends that women have no more than 25 grams of added sugar a day and men have no more than 36 grams of added sugar a day.

TIP

If you want to enjoy a dessert, plan ahead to account for the added calories and sugar in your daily allowance or goals. Or more simply: Save desserts for special occasions and keep the portions small.

The myth that people with diabetes can't eat sweets may stem from the myth that sugar causes type 2 diabetes (see the preceding section). Neither of these myths is true, but perhaps the dangers of too much sugar fuel both misconceptions.

Instead of making certain foods "off limits" to yourself or someone else with diabetes, step back and consider the alternative. Choosing small portions of desserts for special occasions can be healthy for everyone, including those with type 2 diabetes.

Myth 3: People with Diabetes Should Eat Special Diabetic Foods

There are no special "diabetic foods" that people with type 2 diabetes should eat. Healthy food choices and eating strategies are the same for people with or without diabetes. Eating wholesome, nutritious foods is good for you and for everyone else.

You can meet with a dietitian or certified diabetes educator (CDE) if you have questions about what and how much to eat. These professionals can help you develop a meal plan that includes foods you enjoy in appropriate portions. You'll want to consider your goals, lifestyle, and culture when creating a meal plan (see Chapter 12).

It's best to eat a variety of nutritious foods, which are low in saturated fats, added sugars, and refined grains. Nutritious foods include vegetables (of course!), and you can eat nonstarchy vegetables, such as spinach, broccoli, tomatoes, bell peppers, and cucumbers, to your heart's content. They have vitamins, minerals, and fiber — with few calories. Whole grains such as oatmeal, whole-grain bread, and whole-grain pasta have fiber, protein, and essential vitamins and minerals. Fish high in omega-3s such as salmon are good for your heart. (See Chapter 11 for more about healthy eating.)

Foods that people with diabetes should try to avoid include those high in saturated and trans fats, which can raise your cholesterol, clog blood vessels, and put you at greater risk for heart disease, stroke, and other diseases. Try to eat foods with less sodium because sodium can raise blood pressure and increase your risk of cardiovascular, eye, and kidney disease. Avoid added sugar in foods, which are high in calories and low in nutrition.

Some people may think that special "sugar-free" foods are good for people with diabetes, but use caution if you choose to eat these products. Just because a food is labeled "sugar-free" doesn't mean it is carbohydrate free. If it contains carbohydrates, it will still increase your blood glucose. And many sugar-free foods contain sugar alcohols that can cause gastrointestinal pain and even diarrhea when eaten in large quantities. Your best bet is to stick with nutrient-rich foods as often as possible.

Myth 4: People with Diabetes Are More Likely to Get a Cold or the Flu

You are not more likely to get a cold or the flu if you have diabetes. As far as cold season goes, you're just as lucky or as unlucky as anyone else walking around on a drizzly, cold February day.

However, you should get an annual flu shot to help protect against influenza. People with diabetes can have more serious complications of the flu and can go on to develop pneumonia. The flu also makes managing your blood glucose a pain because it can affect those numbers.

REMEMBER

It's still possible to get the flu even if you've had a flu shot. But you'll probably have a less severe reaction to the flu virus than if you'd had no shot at all.

The best way to prevent colds and the flu is the same for people with and without diabetes:

» Wash your hands frequently and encourage your children or spouse to do the same.

» Keep germs to yourself by using tissues or asking kids to sneeze or cough into their elbows so they avoid getting germs on their hands.

» Try to avoid hanging out with other people who have colds, although that can be hard when it's your spouse sleeping next to you or a sick child resting on your lap!

» Keep your body and mind in tip-top shape to avoid infections. Eat healthy foods, exercise, and get plenty of sleep. Also, try to minimize stress (flip back to Chapter 14 for tips on handling stress).

Myth 5: You've Failed If Your Doctor Says You Need to Start Taking Insulin

This myth is damaging because it's untrue and hurtful to people with diabetes. Many people with type 2 diabetes use insulin, and it's not because they failed or didn't take the right steps.

In fact, people often feel frustrated not just because they need to start taking insulin, but because they need to change medications frequently. For example, you may have started your diabetes treatment by taking metformin, but in the years since you've added certain medications or switched to another medication altogether.

The reason behind these changes is that type 2 diabetes is a *progressive disease.* People with type 2 diabetes may still be able to produce insulin, the hormone necessary to turn the food we eat into fuel for our bodies. However, your cells may not produce enough insulin, or they may not be as sensitive to insulin — probably both.

Over months and years, your cells work overtime to make up for that loss of insulin, and they burn out. It's a progression — and the progression isn't the same for each person with diabetes. Some people may have a swift progression, and other people may have a slower progression in the decline of those insulin-making cells.

Therefore, some people may stick to the same medication over a long period of time because it works. Meanwhile, other people need to switch medications and perhaps start insulin because other medications are no longer effective.

Psychologically, you may feel like you failed because you feel the effects of this progression — and feel responsible. Try to keep those thoughts at bay because they're not true and not helpful.

TIP

Instead, try to focus on learning all you can about insulin and how to use it (see Chapter 6). Using insulin is different from taking a pill, so you may feel overwhelmed at first by the new routine. Don't worry. Your physician, nurse, or diabetes educator can help you get started and answer questions along the way. Check out an online support group where you'll find other people with type 2 diabetes voicing similar questions and concerns about starting insulin (see Chapter 14 for advice on finding a support group).

Myth 6: Diabetes Is Not That Serious of a Disease

Diabetes causes more deaths a year than breast cancer and AIDS combined. It affects individuals and families and businesses and schools. By 2050, one out of three Americans could have diabetes, if current trends continue, according to the Centers for Disease Control and Prevention.

Sometimes type 2 diabetes may not seem serious because it often develops without symptoms. It may seem like you can ignore it and deal with it later. However, this thinking is part of the reason why diabetes can be so devastating. The long-term effects of high blood glucose can damage your body and increase your risk for heart disease, stroke, kidney failure, blindness, and amputations.

However, you can reduce your risk of complications by recognizing that diabetes is a serious disease. The good news is that you can take active steps to improve your blood glucose by losing weight, eating healthy foods, exercising, and taking your medications. These steps truly work!

6

Standing Up for Yourself

Navigate the ins and outs of health insurance coverage of diabetes medications and supplies.

Find out what questions to ask before surgery and hospital stays.

Discover your rights in the workplace.

Plan ahead for travel and get through airport security with ease.

» Knowing where you can get insurance

» Finding help when you don't have insurance

» Preparing for other healthcare scenarios

Chapter **18**

Navigating Health Insurance and Other Healthcare Scenarios

Health insurance is a hot-button topic that weighs on everyone's mind and impacts everyone's wallet. Most Americans have differing opinions about how it should work — including who and what it should cover. But everyone can agree on one thing: Access to healthcare, medications, and supplies keeps getting more expensive.

People with diabetes should have access to health insurance because it helps them afford medications (including insulin), blood glucose meters, test strips, and insulin supplies. It also allows people with diabetes to visit their healthcare providers for preventive care, routine management, and treatment for life-threatening complications of diabetes.

In this chapter, we give you the lay of the land in terms of the health insurance marketplace, including protections that specifically affect people with type 2 diabetes. These things can change quickly, so stay informed by visiting www. diabetes.org or www.healthcare.gov for updates. You also find tips for finding diabetes care and supplies if you don't have health insurance. Finally, we give you some specifics on hospital stays, home healthcare, and long-term care.

Protecting People with Diabetes

The Affordable Care Act (ACA), also called Obamacare, was passed in 2010 and afforded Americans — particularly people with diabetes and their families — new health insurance protections.

This protection could change if the ACA is repealed or significantly modified. Whatever happens, it's important to know how the landscape of health insurance changed for people with diabetes with this act.

Under the ACA, people with preexisting conditions such as diabetes cannot be denied health insurance coverage or charged a higher premium. This is true for both employer-based plans and individual plans. Also, plans cannot cancel insurance policies for people because they're diagnosed with diabetes or other conditions.

Also, young adults can stay on their parents' health insurance until they're 26 years old under the ACA, so children with diabetes don't need to worry about losing their health insurance until they're in their mid-20s.

Free preventive care also changed under the ACA because all plans are required to offer it. As a general rule, preventive care covers diabetes screening for adults with certain risk factors or pregnant women. It might cover obesity and high cholesterol screening. Medicare also covers specific preventive care programs for people with diabetes, which we outline later in this chapter.

The ACA also mandated that health insurance plans cover "essential health benefits" such as medications, chronic disease management, and hospitalization — and plans can't put a cap on how much they'll pay for these benefits each calendar year or during a person's lifetime while enrolled in that plan. The details of these benefits vary by plan and by state, so it's important to do your homework when shopping for plans.

One more thing under ACA: Anyone can request an easy-to-read explanation of his benefits from his health insurance company. It's called a Summary of Benefits of Coverage (SBC). For instance, you can ask for an example of how the plan might cover a typical patient with type 2 diabetes.

Understanding Health Insurance: Employer, Government, and Individual

Health insurance is offered through three primary channels in the United States today. You can get health insurance through your employer, you can qualify for government-based health insurance such as Medicare or Medicaid, or you can buy health insurance on your own. The following sections tell you what you need to know about each form of insurance.

Employer-based health insurance

Your employer may offer health insurance to its employees; many people are familiar with this type of insurance. The coverage is usually offered for you and your spouse and dependents.

Employer-based health insurance is not the same across all companies. Large companies may offer their employees several health insurance plans to choose from. Small companies may only offer one insurance plan (and some very small companies offer none). Small businesses can buy insurance through a program called the Small Business Health Options Program (SHOP) marketplace, which can make health insurance more affordable.

REMEMBER

Generic drugs are cheaper than brand-name drugs, so ask your pharmacist or provider about whether a generic version could be a cost-saving option. This also goes for diabetes supplies like meters and test strips. Switching to a store-brand version could save you money.

Government-based health insurance

Medicare, Medicaid, and the U.S. Department of Veterans Affairs provide health insurance for many Americans. Important coverage for people with diabetes is included within government programs, so read on for more details.

Medicare

Medicare is the federal program that provides health insurance for millions of Americans 65 years of age or older. It also provides health insurance to people with certain disabilities and people with end-stage kidney disease. Medicare is run by the Centers for Medicare and Medicaid Services, which is part of the U.S. Department of Health and Human Services.

You'll still have to make co-pays and pay for certain services or medications under Medicare. Check out www.medicare.gov for more details.

Medicare is broken down into different parts (A, B, C, D, and Medigap), and you've probably heard these terms mentioned on the news or during commercials. You're not dreaming if you think Medicare is complicated. It's a large government program that has specific rules and coverage. And it's been around (and modified plenty) for the past 50 years. Here's a breakdown of what each part covers:

>> **Medicare Part A:** Medicare Part A covers hospital costs, including skilled nursing facilities, hospice, and some home healthcare.

>> **Medicare Part B:** Medicare Part B covers medical costs, including visits to your diabetes care provider, medical equipment and supplies, diagnostic tests, and outpatient visits to a hospital or physical therapy. Part B is important for people with diabetes because it covers things like blood glucose meters, test strips, and lancets. It also covers preventive care such as tests for diabetes, cardiovascular disease, obesity, and eye disease. It covers diabetes education and nutrition therapy.

Medicare Part B covers the following services for diabetes:

- Diabetes education (10 hours at diagnosis and up to 2 hours yearly)

- Dilated eye exam

- Foot exam

- Glaucoma test

- Medical nutrition therapy

Coverage for these services can vary so ask your provider for details.

Medicare Part B covers the following supplies for diabetes:

- Blood glucose meters, control solution, and test strips. Continuous glucose monitors (CGMs) may also be covered depending on the manufacturer.

- Insulin pumps (and pump insulin), if medically necessary

- Lancet devices and lancets

- Therapeutic shoes or inserts

You may have to buy these supplies from certain suppliers for coverage under Medicare Part B. Also Medicare offers a national mail-order program for diabetes supplies. For more information on this mail-order program visit www.medicare.gov/what-medicare-covers/part-b/dme-diabetes-national-mail-order-program.html.

>> **Medicare Part C:** Medicare Part C is actually a system of Medicare Advantage plans, which are private health plans. They cover Part A, Part B, and sometimes Part D in one package. It's a different way of receiving Medicare benefits than traditional Medicare. You can find more details about these plans at www.medicare.gov.

>> **Medicare Part D:** Medicare Part D covers prescription drugs like pills for blood glucose and insulin supplies. You buy a Part D plan and pay a separate premium and co-pays for your medication. Each plan may cover different medications or brands, so take your time to review plans before making a decision.

Medicare Part D plans usually cover the following supplies for diabetes:

- Blood glucose medications

- Syringes, needles, and alcohol swabs

- Insulin (not given through a pump)

>> **Medigap:** Medigap is private insurance that covers the extra costs of Medicare such as co-pays and deductibles.

Medicare can be confusing. For more details about this complicated government insurance, check out *Medicare For Dummies*, 2nd Edition, by Patricia Barry (Wiley).

Medicaid and CHIP

Medicaid and the Children's Health Insurance Program (CHIP) provide health coverage for millions of low-income Americans and their families, and those with disabilities. Medicaid is a joint federal and state program; you can find out more on your state's Medicaid website or at www.medicaid.gov.

CHIP provides low-cost health insurance for children and teens whose families can't afford employer-based or individual health insurance, but whose incomes are too high to qualify for Medicaid. Pregnant women may qualify, too. Go to www.insurekidsnow.gov to find out more about this program.

TRICARE

TRICARE is a healthcare program for active-duty and retired service members and their families. Go to www.tricare.mil to find out about eligibility and coverage for diabetes medical care and supplies. The U.S. Department of Veterans Affairs provides healthcare for veterans. Go to www.va.gov for more info.

TIP

Some states have Consumer Assistance Programs that can help people with concerns about health insurance and claims: www.healthcare.gov/how-can-i-get-consumer-help-if-i-have-insurance.

Individual health insurance

You may need to purchase your own health insurance if you're unemployed, if you're self-employed, or if you don't qualify for the government-based insurance plans explained in the preceding section. You can buy individual and family health insurance plans on health insurance marketplaces or exchanges. And you buy this plan in your state; some states such as Colorado and California run their own marketplaces, while other states such as Georgia and Hawaii rely on the federal government to run these marketplaces. Visit www.healthcare.gov to find your state's marketplace. You can also buy individual and family health insurance plans directly from insurance companies.

Fill out an application on the marketplace to find out your health insurance plan options. This will also tell you whether you qualify for government programs such as Medicaid and CHIP or whether you qualify for financial assistance. You can enroll or change plans in the fall or winter for coverage in January of the following year. Certain life events like losing your job, changing your marital status, or having a baby will allow you to change plans at different times.

Coverage for diabetes medication and services varies from plan to plan on the individual marketplace. It's up to you as the consumer to compare the price of premiums, deductibles, medications, and diabetes supplies.

Everyone with health insurance has likely been denied coverage for a service or medication that they thought would be paid for. It feels terrible. And it can be very expensive, too.

TIP

Don't be shy about filing a claim (also called an *appeal*) once, twice, or even three times. You may need to ask your provider to write a letter on your behalf explaining why you need a particular medication or a particular device like a continuous glucose monitor or an insulin pen as opposed to a syringe (which may be easier for people with dexterity issues). You may also need to write your own letter and provide records.

Asking the Right Questions

Choosing the right insurance coverage, especially when you have a chronic disease like diabetes, can be difficult and frustrating. To help make this process a little easier, the following sections detail questions to ask about diabetes coverage when selecting an insurance plan and questions to ask to determine which plan is right for you.

Questions to ask about diabetes coverage

When considering what insurance plan to sign up for, make sure you compare apples to apples as best you can. Use the following questions to understand how different insurance companies cover diabetes care:

>> How many times can I see my diabetes care provider each year?

>> Can I see a provider of my choice or will it cost extra?

>> How much will I have to pay each visit?

>> Does the plan allow me to see a specialist of my choice — such as a podiatrist or dermatologist? Will I need a referral from my primary care physician? And how much extra might it cost?

>> Are eye exams covered? How much will they cost?

>> Does the plan cover mental health, such as sessions with a therapist?

>> Which prescriptions are covered? What's the co-pay, and does the company offer a prescription plan to reduce costs?

>> Does the plan cover blood glucose meters, strips, syringes, pens, or other necessary supplies? Which brands and how many each month?

>> Does the plan cover insulin pumps and continuous glucose monitors for people with type 2 diabetes?

>> Does the plan cover diabetes education and medical nutrition therapy? How many hours?

TIP

Sometimes plans offer tiers of coverage for different medications. When comparing plans, make a list of your current medications and see where they fall in the coverage tier. Add up these co-pays to determine your monthly outlay for medications.

You can ask your provider or pharmacist for assistance in determining coverage for your medication under your plan.

General questions to ask about plans

Use the following questions to choose an insurance plan that best suits your needs:

>> How much will the plan cost each year?

>> What is the deductible? In other words, how much do I have to pay before I get coverage?

>> After I've met my deductible, how much will I pay for services?

>> What is the co-pay for different services?

>> Which doctors can I see as part of my plan?

>> Which hospitals can I go to as part of my plan?

>> Is home healthcare or long-term care included?

Finding Help for People Who Don't Have Insurance

Some people can't afford or don't have access to health insurance. People with diabetes who are uninsured need assistance paying for basic and specialty care, prescriptions, and supplies. The following sections can help you obtain the care you need.

Primary and specialty care for the uninsured

The Bureau of Primary Health Care oversees a network of community health centers that offer free and sliding-scale services for people who can't afford medical care. Visit www.bphc.hrsa.gov to find a community health center in your area.

EyeCare America (www.aao.org/eyecare-america) and VISION USA (www.aoafoundation.org/vision-usa) offer free eye exams to low-income and uninsured people. Also, the Patient Access Network Foundation (www.panfoundation.org) offers help with payments for certain treatments and medications that patients can't afford.

Prescriptions for the uninsured

Partnership for Prescription Assistance (www.pparx.org) helps people find free or low-cost medications by partnering with pharmaceutical companies, doctors, and other groups. Simplefill (www.simplefill.com) is another program that helps patients find low-cost medications.

RxAssist (www.rxassist.org) and NeedyMeds (www.needymeds.org) have websites where you can search for prescription assistance programs.

These are just a few of the programs out there, and the American Diabetes Association doesn't endorse any particular program. Pharmaceutical companies may also offer their own patient assistance programs for those in need.

Diabetes supplies for the uninsured

Rx Outreach (www.rxoutreach.org) is a nonprofit mail-order pharmacy offering diabetes medications and supplies at a discounted price. CR3 Diabetes Association offers discounted supplies such as pumps, meters, and tests strips (www.cr3diabetes.org). The National Council on Aging also offers a tool for searching for programs that could save you money (www.benefitscheckup.org).

Anticipating Other Healthcare Scenarios

Regular checkups aren't the only time that you'll see doctors and nurses. You may check into the emergency room or hospital or need home care or long-term care.

Your diabetes may not be the thing that prompts you to check into the hospital or decide on a skilled nursing home. In fact, it could be for something completely different like a fall or pneumonia or just not feeling safe living alone. Nevertheless, consider your diabetes when navigating these different scenarios. In this section, you find tips and action steps to take when being admitted to a hospital or long-term-care center or receiving healthcare (such as physical therapy or dialysis) in your own home.

ER visits and hospital stays

No one wants to go to the hospital or emergency room, but inevitably you may find yourself there some day or evening (perhaps even at midnight). Sometimes a hospital visit is easy to predict, like when you have a scheduled surgery. Other times, it's unexpected, like when you slip on that nasty patch of ice going to the mailbox.

Emergency room visits

The number-one thing to remember when you find yourself in the emergency room (ER) is to tell the doctors and nurses that you have type 2 diabetes. Then tell them about any other conditions such as eye disease or high blood pressure. Also, be sure to tell them if you frequently experience episodes of low blood glucose and describe your own personal symptoms. Don't be embarrassed. You may not be able to tell a nurse these things when you're actually experiencing a low. (See more about lows in Chapter 8.)

Consider wearing a medical ID bracelet to inform first responders and ER staff that you have type 2 diabetes. This could be important if you're unconscious for some reason. Order ID bracelets (from fashion to sport versions) at www.shopdiabetes.org, other online retailers, or your local pharmacy. You can engrave bracelets with your name, the words *type 2 diabetes,* an emergency contact number, or essential medications like insulin.

Planned hospital stays

If your hospital stay is scheduled, ask the hospital staff how they'll help you manage your blood glucose during your stay. For example, the staff will probably monitor your blood glucose during your stay so you may not need to worry about bringing your meter or test strips to the hospital. However, specifically ask the hospital staff how they plan to monitor blood glucose and whether to bring your meter. You may also stop taking diabetes pills and switch to insulin during your stay.

Your physical activity and food probably won't be the same. You may not be able to do all the things that you normally do, so come up with a plan for your hospital stay. If the hospital has a dietitian on staff, you can ask to speak to that person. Ideally, you'll be able to keep your blood glucose in your target range, which will help you get healthy faster and reduce the risk of complications.

TIP

Consider asking your diabetes care provider about which hospital she recommends in your area. You may only have one hospital in town, but if you have alternatives, it's helpful to know the most respected facility for caring for people with diabetes.

Scheduled surgery

If you're having a surgery that your doctor schedules ahead of time, you'll have more time to plan ahead for your hospital stay. Ask your doctor how to best prepare for your upcoming procedure. For example, she may recommend that you have your blood glucose in a certain range. You may also need to stop taking certain medications like blood thinners. Ask whether you'll need to tweak your insulin regimen beforehand or temporarily withhold any blood glucose medications.

TIP

Tell the surgeon and the anesthesiologist that you have type 2 diabetes, and give them a list of all the medications that you take for diabetes and any other conditions. Ask how your blood glucose will be managed during surgery.

Going home: The good and the bad

Getting discharged from the hospital and going home is wonderful. You might be able to sleep in your own bed again or eat your favorite snack. But it can also make some people nervous, especially if they're worried about taking care of themselves or managing a new regimen.

The hospital should provide detailed instructions about how to take care of yourself, including changes to your diabetes care routine. However, you may consider calling your diabetes care provider, diabetes educator, or another member of your team to follow up. You can also ask them questions, talk about concerns, or schedule an appointment for a checkup.

Home healthcare and long-term care

Home healthcare is an option if you need help taking care of yourself but want to stay in your own home. Sometimes this could happen when you get discharged from the hospital but you still need to do physical therapy or receive care. Sometimes people with type 2 diabetes and kidney failure have dialysis treatments at home.

Several home healthcare agencies provide these services, so check with your health insurance about coverage. Ask for recommendations on these agencies from your diabetes care team and friends and family.

TIP

When comparing health insurance plans, don't forget to look at coverage for home healthcare. Home healthcare is often covered under Medicare, but check your benefits, too.

You may need long-term care if you go to a rehabilitation center or specialty hospital. *Long-term care* can also refer to a skilled nursing facility or nursing home where doctors and nurses are available 24/7. Choosing these centers is not always easy, so ask for recommendations from people you trust.

TIP

If you can, visit the facilities ahead of time and bring a friend or family member for their insight. You can find resources at www.eldercare.gov and compare nursing homes at www.medicare.gov. Hospital discharge planners and social workers can also help.

WARNING

Long-term care is not always covered under health insurance, and sometimes it's not fully covered. You can purchase long-term-care insurance to plan for your needs down the road.

Chapter **19**

Knowing Your Rights

You may spend a big chunk of your day at work, or your child may spend most of her days at school. So, it's important to consider diabetes management in these situations and make sure you create the best environment for success. You have certain rights as a person with diabetes, and we detail them in this chapter. We also talk about how to keep those rights in mind when starting a new job, telling your co-workers or boss about your diabetes, or designing a safe and successful learning plan for your child with diabetes.

Travel is another activity that you can plan for in terms of your diabetes supplies, medications, and management of your blood glucose. In this chapter, find out about Transportation Security Administration (TSA) regulations, as well as tips for taking road trips or other types of vacations.

REMEMBER

The American Diabetes Association is dedicated to helping you understand and advocate for your rights as a person with diabetes. People with diabetes have many legal protections, but there is still more work to be done. Keep in mind that ignorance may be one of the most common affronts you experience as a person with diabetes or as a parent of a child with diabetes. Knowing your rights can help you navigate (and perhaps defuse) these situations so you can educate other people about diabetes and, ultimately, create a successful work or learning environment. It's not always easy or fair to have a chronic condition such as diabetes. We have tips to help you manage your diabetes and talk to others about it — whether you're on the job, in school, or at the airport.

Diabetes in the Workplace

Whether you're starting a new job or you've been at your company for years, you'll want to consider your diabetes management at your workplace. Some things to think about include who (if anyone) to tell about your diabetes and how to communicate and educate others. You'll want to know your rights and responsibilities as someone with diabetes.

Deciding whether to tell others

Your first question about diabetes at work is probably: Should I tell anyone? Well, it's generally up to you.

You may want to tell people about your diabetes for various reasons. For example, you may have a rigorous job that makes it difficult to take sudden breaks for blood glucose checks or to give an insulin injection. Telling your co-workers and boss could make those self-care breaks go more smoothly. Or you may be concerned about low blood glucose emergencies. In this case, you can tell co-workers how to help in an emergency if they volunteer, including information about where you keep your glucagon and the importance of calling 911.

Some people with diabetes don't feel comfortable sharing personal information about their health. Others may work from home or have a flexible environment that makes self-care more private and relaxed.

TIP

Sometimes a potential employer will make a conditional job offer that requires the employee to complete a pre-employment physical. In this situation, you'd be required to disclose that you have diabetes. And the employer could withdraw the offer if you don't comply. It's important to note that an employer may not request any disability-related information or give any medical examinations *prior* to making a job offer to the applicant.

Talking about your diabetes in the workplace really is a personal decision that's up to you. In the following section, find out about your rights so you can make an informed decision about talking about diabetes on the job.

Knowing your rights

People with diabetes are protected against discrimination by disability laws. It may seem strange to think of yourself as someone with a disability, but your diabetes is a disability because it limits the endocrine system. You probably manage your diabetes with medications or lifestyle changes or both. However, your diabetes still qualifies as a disability because the law considers how a person would be if he stopped managing or treating his diabetes.

Several federal, state, and local laws protect people with disabilities, including people with diabetes. Usually federal and state protections are similar, but in states where disability laws are stronger, those state protections supersede any federal protections. And in states where the federal law is stronger than the state law, the federal law applies. Call 800-DIABETES (800-342-2383) for more information on your state's anti-discrimination laws.

Here's a rundown of the federal anti-discrimination laws you should be aware of:

>> **Americans with Disabilities Act:** Protects employees against discrimination by private employers, labor unions, employment agencies, and state and local governments.

>> **Rehabilitation Act of 1973:** Protects employees against discrimination in federal employment, and in the employment practices of federal contractors and employers that receive federal money.

>> **Americans with Disabilities Act Amendments Act of 2008:** Amends the Americans with Disabilities Act and the Rehabilitation Act of 1973 by expanding the definition of the term *disability*, making it clear that people with diabetes are protected from discrimination in the workplace.

>> **Congressional Accountability Act:** Protects employees of Congress and its Legislative Branch agencies.

REMEMBER

The Family Medical Leave Act (FMLA) allows you up to 12 weeks of time off work (unpaid) to care for your own serious health condition, such as diabetes, or to care for a family member with diabetes. You can take this leave in small blocks of time such as 1-hour increments.

Not all employers are covered under the FMLA. The act applies to all public agencies, all public and private elementary and secondary schools, and companies with 50 or more employees. Also, it can only be used to care for an immediate family member (spouse, child, or parent).

What are my protections?

Under disability laws (see the preceding section), your employer can't discriminate against you because of your diabetes. You may experience discrimination in any number of circumstances such as hiring, while on the job, in training, promotions, tenure, and leaves of absence. If you have questions or think you may have experienced discrimination, call the American Diabetes Association at 800-DIABETES (800-342-2383). The American Diabetes Association can provide information and assistance to better understand your rights.

Some key protections under the law:

>> Your employer can't refuse to hire or promote you because of your diabetes.

>> Your employer can't fire you because of your diabetes unless you pose a "direct threat" or can no longer perform the essential functions of your job with reasonable accommodations.

>> Your employer must provide reasonable accommodations that help you perform the essential functions of the job.

>> Your employer must not discriminate against you for health insurance offered in the workplace because of your diabetes.

For more specifics about these protections, visit www.diabetes.org or call the American Diabetes Association advocacy team at 800-DIABETES (800-342-2383).

Educating and communicating with others

If you decide to tell others about your diabetes, take a moment beforehand to think about what you want to say. You may want to be fairly succinct and straight-forward, telling people that you have diabetes and that you manage it on your own. However, in an emergency during hypoglycemia, you may need their help finding your glucagon or calling 911.

Check out the Centers for Disease Control and Prevention's program Diabetes at Work by visiting www.cdc.gov/diabetes/diabetesatwork. It has resources about the prevention and management of diabetes in the workplace, including wellness programs, fact sheets, and best practices for helping employees manage their diabetes at work.

Consider keeping an extra supply of glucagon at your desk or workplace so you'll have it on hand if you have a low.

Staying healthy on the job

Many companies now offer wellness programs for employees, so take advantage of these benefits. Your employer may offer discounts for gym memberships or offer in-house exercise programs such as yoga classes. Some health insurance plans reward policyholders for exercise if they meet fitness goals while wearing their fitness trackers.

Stress is an all too common component of the workplace, and stress can affect blood glucose. Check your blood glucose if you're concerned about it for any reason, and keep in mind that your mental health is important on the job, too. Check out Chapter 14 for more strategies to manage stress.

If you have a desk job, remember to stand up and take breaks throughout the day. The American Diabetes Association recommends that people with type 2 diabetes get up every 30 minutes for 3–4 minutes of activity such as arm stretches or walking in place. Take a walk down the hall, or better yet, take the stairs down and walk around the building before taking the stairs back up to your desk. (Flip to Chapter 13 for more information about sitting less and moving more.)

Your Child with Diabetes at School

Your child will spend the majority of her day at school, so you'll need to work together with school administrators, the school nurse, and other school staff to ensure he is safe and successful. Your school may not be familiar with caring for and supporting preteens and teens with type 2 diabetes. After all, the increase of type 2 diabetes in young people is a fairly recent health concern. Don't be discouraged. Take the opportunity to educate others about diabetes and advocate for your child. He may need special accommodations during the school day so he can be a safe, healthy, and successful student.

Knowing and advocating for your child's rights

Children with diabetes are protected against discrimination by disability laws. It may be hard to think of your child as having a disability, but diabetes is a disability because it limits the function of the endocrine system. Students with diabetes have the right to enroll and participate in school just like any other students. They have the right to take care of their diabetes and be safe, as well as have the opportunity to learn.

Federal laws protect children with diabetes at school, and some state laws give further protections and clarification about which school staff are allowed to provide diabetes care. Go to www.diabetes.org/kidswin to find specific information on your state's laws and read on for information on federal laws.

Section 504 of the federal Rehabilitation Act of 1973 is a federal anti-discrimination law that protects children in public schools and private and religious schools that receive federal funding. It requires schools to provide needed diabetes care and services and to treat children with diabetes fairly, so they may participate in all school-sponsored activities. Students who are able to self-manage should be allowed to do so anywhere, anytime. Having written accommodations plans like a 504 Plan helps ensure that your child's diabetes needs are met in school (see the following section for details on 504 Plans).

The Americans with Disabilities Act also protects people with disabilities such as diabetes, and applies to public schools, private schools, camps, and other programs (except those run by religious institutions).

The Individuals with Disabilities Education Act is another federal law that gives states money to help provide education and services for children with disabilities like diabetes. Children whose diabetes or other disability interferes with learning and academic progress are eligible for services under this law.

REMEMBER

The FMLA allows you up to 12 weeks of time off work (unpaid) to care for an immediate family member such as a child with diabetes, if your employer is a public entity or has 50 or more employees. For example, you could take this time to respond to a diabetes-related emergency at school or if your child is newly diagnosed or hospitalized. You can take this leave in small blocks of time, even as small as 1-hour increments.

Putting care plans in writing

A *Diabetes Medical Management Plan* (DMMP) can help your child receive the care she needs at school or camp. You work with your doctor to detail your child's diabetes care needs at school, such as times to check blood glucose, following a diabetes meal plan, physical activity, and how to handle emergencies.

TIP

Templates for a DMMP can be found online at www.diabetes.org/dmmp, but your child's provider may need to tweak it based on your child's specific needs and health.

A written accommodations plan, like a 504 Plan, is different. It details how your child can stay safe by receiving needed care, self-managing his diabetes, and participating fully in school. It may include provisions such as permission to make extra trips to the bathroom or offering non-food rewards and providing healthy foods for class parties. It may outline training for staff to understand diabetes. It may set aside alternate arrangements for making up missed assignments and exams, time missed for medical appointments, or other issues related to diabetes. You can find sample 504 Plans online at www.diabetes.org/504plan.

TIP

Educate yourself before you take action. Visit www.diabetes.org/safeatschool or call 800-DIABETES (800-342-2383) to find out more about your child's rights at school and how to make sure your child gets needed care at school.

Planning Ahead for Travel

Your diabetes shouldn't slow you down from traveling, whether you're off for a long weekend or a month-long European vacation. You'll want to plan ahead by talking to your physician, bringing extra medication, preparing for airport security if needed, and thinking about snacks and meals.

Talking to your physician

If you're planning a longer vacation, talk to your healthcare provider about what you'll need to take care of your diabetes while you're away from home. Ask about precautions to take before you leave or considerations while you're on your trip.

Your physician may recommend that you bring extra medication on your travels. Determine whether you have enough or whether you'll need new prescriptions before you hit the road.

REMEMBER

If you use insulin, you'll want to plan ahead for how you'll store your insulin safely and in a cool place during your travels. Also, plan ahead for a portable way to dispose of syringes. You can find handy insulin storage and syringe disposal tools online.

Preparing for airport security

Going through security at the airport is sometimes a hassle, but it shouldn't be more of a hassle because of diabetes. Here's the skinny on how to get through the checkpoint with minimal hiccups.

The American Diabetes Association works with the Transportation Security Administration (TSA) to make sure people with diabetes have access to their supplies and equipment as they go through security checkpoints and board their plane. It's always a good idea to arrive 2–3 hours early, pack diabetes supplies and medication in a clear plastic bag, and make sure to bring extra supplies. Most people can bring 3.4 ounces or less of liquids through security. However, people with diabetes can exceed those limits with medications, including insulin and glucagon, or drinks for treating a low such as juice.

REMEMBER

If you use insulin, take it through security instead of placing it in your checked bag where it's subject to extreme temperatures and pressure (and could get delayed or lost if your bag doesn't end up in the same place you do).

TIP

TSA Cares is a helpline designed to assist travelers with disabilities like diabetes. Travelers seeking assistance should call 855-787-2227 at least 72 hours in advance. An optional Disability Notification Card, which you can print out online at www.tsa.com is a quick (and discreet) way to inform screeners about your diabetes. More information can be found at www.diabetes.org/airtravel.

Considering snacks and meals out

Your travel may put you on a different meal schedule than normal, so you may want to pack snacks to avoid low blood glucose. Raisins, energy bars, or glucose tablets are easy to have on hand.

You may also eat out more if you're on the road, and eating healthy foods may be more challenging because you're not cooking in your own kitchen. Think ahead about healthy options such as a simple breakfast in your hotel room or fast-food restaurants that offer nutritious, low-sodium meals. (See Chapter 12 for more tips on eating out.)

TIP

You may want to check your blood glucose more often when you're on vacation if you're on an irregular eating schedule or you're more active than usual.

Taking care of your feet and skin

Pay attention to your feet when you're on vacation to prevent problems that could interfere later in the trip or when you return home. Your feet may swell when you fly, and compression socks can help. You may walk more than usual on vacation (a great thing!), so pack comfortable shoes and breathable socks. If you have foot problems, try not to go barefoot on the sand or riverbank. Hot sand, shells on the beach, or other sharp debris can create small cuts that may be hard to feel if you have neuropathy or may take a long time to heal. Instead, buy a pair of comfortable waterproof sandals or shoes.

Wear sunscreen and put on a hat if you're traveling someplace sunny or at high elevation. Cracked or peeling skin may become infected, so it's best to prevent sunburns in the first place. Also, some diabetes medications such as glipizide and glyburide can make you more sensitive to the sun. The sun's rays can be powerful, and it's easy to forget to reapply sunscreen if you haven't been at the beach for a while.

Ensuring Safety while Driving

Generally, people with diabetes aren't restricted when driving or getting a private driver's license. There may be some restrictions for obtaining a commercial driver's license. All states have special licensing rules about medical conditions. Some states apply these rules to all drivers with diabetes. Others apply them only to people with certain medications or symptoms (insulin use, loss of consciousness, low blood glucose, seizures, foot problems such as neuropathy, and vision problems such as retinopathy).

Follow the same safety guidelines as others when driving your car, such as not drinking alcohol or using drugs while driving. Consider your blood glucose if you're feeling low or experiencing more lows than usual. Carry your blood glucose meter and glucose tablets or gels. Be aware of warning signs of low blood glucose (see Chapter 8), and pull over if you feel a low coming on.

Some people with diabetes may have complications such as vision problems or sensation problems related to nerves or blood vessels in their hands or feet. Talk with your healthcare provider about whether these complications may affect your driving, and ask for a referral to a driving specialist who can evaluate your driving.

7

The Part of Tens

IN THIS PART . . .

Inject fun into your fitness routine by adding music, an exercise buddy, or both.

Keep tabs on your blood glucose, blood pressure, and cholesterol for excellent eye health.

Chapter **20**

Ten Fun Ways to Work Out for People Who Hate to Exercise

Exercise is one of the best things you can do for your diabetes. The benefits are enormous. It can improve your mood and fight depression. It actually makes your body more sensitive to insulin and lowers blood glucose. It also improves cholesterol and blood pressure levels. And you could lose a few pounds to look and feel better, too.

If exercise is so good, why aren't we all exercising every single chance we get? Because exercise can be difficult. It's not easy to stay motivated, especially if you've been sedentary, you're overweight, or you have pain in your joints. It's not easy to find the time if you're working all day and then trying to take care of your kids or your aging parents at night. It's not easy if your neighborhood is unsafe or the temperature is extremely hot or cold.

Despite these obstacles, there are proven strategies for getting more physically fit. One of the best things you can do is choose exercise that you enjoy and that's fun! Exercise and fun — those two words might not go together for many people. But you might be surprised by how thrilling exercise can be if you choose activities that appeal to you.

In this chapter, you discover how to take new steps to get more physically active — and how to inject some joy in those steps.

Get a Buddy

No matter what type of exercise you choose, it's usually more fun to do it with someone else. Why? Well, humans are innately social animals. We like to talk and connect and share our experiences with others. It fights feelings of isolation — and encourages our engagement with our family, friends, neighbors, and the larger community.

You might choose a friend, a co-worker, a spouse, or your kid to be an exercise buddy. It all depends on what kind of physical activity you select and whether that person is interested in joining you. Choose someone who is just as interested in exercising as you are — or, even better, *more* interested. That way, when you feel unmotivated or tired, your buddy can encourage you to get moving. Don't be intimidated about asking someone to join you in exercise.

TIP

Schedule the exercise with your buddy ahead of time. That way, you'll both have it on your calendar, and you won't be as likely to ditch exercise because other things come up. Having someone else make a commitment to your exercise goals can be a powerful thing.

Talking with a buddy while you exercise, whether walking on the treadmill at the gym or taking a brisk walk during your lunch breaks, can take your mind off the difficulty of the exercise. You might get distracted by talking or hearing about someone else's day and forget that you didn't feel like exercising in the first place. Hey, this is a time when gossiping is actually a good thing!

Play like a Kid

There's a reason kids are the best exercisers around: They don't even think it's exercise. For kids, playing soccer or climbing to the top of the jungle gym isn't a way to burn calories. It's just fun!

We could all take a lesson from kids by looking at exercise through the same rose-colored glasses. Instead of stressing that you don't have time to go to the gym this week, just ask your kids or your grandkids to play. You might be surprised by what they come up with. You could find yourself on a bike ride — but you might also find yourself tossing a Frisbee or playing duck-duck-goose or hide and seek.

Never underestimate the ability of a good pillow fight to bring contagious grins to everyone's faces.

If you don't have any kids around to bring out your inner child, try thinking about your favorite things that you did as a kid. Maybe you liked to swim or take walks in the woods or play Ping-Pong. Don't look at your watch; just immerse yourself in these activities that give you pleasure.

Start Walking

It may sound too simple, but walking is one of the best ways to get exercise. Why? Because it's so easy for almost everyone to do. You don't need a fancy gym or fancy shoes — or even oodles of time. The freedom to walk can be fun because it's possible for almost everyone.

Look at your day as a way to incorporate more steps. One way to make it fun (and a challenge) is to wear a pedometer or fitness tracker to measure your steps. For example, you might enjoy using a Fitbit, but there are less expensive versions out there, too. You might start by walking for just 10 minutes a day because you haven't been physically active in a while. Or you might be ready to start walking for 30 minutes in the morning before work. The steps in between exercise are just as important. You might start taking the stairs in your apartment building or walking your dog for 5 minutes longer.

TIP

Taking even a 10-minute walk, specifically after your evening meal, could improve your blood glucose, according to a small study of 41 people with type 2 diabetes published in 2016.

There's an App (or Video) for That

Finding fun in exercise has never been easier thanks to new mobile apps and online videos. You can stream videos of exercise classes on your phone, iPad, or computer. For example, you can stream yoga or strength-training videos or even a video of hiking through the desert. But really, the joy of apps and online videos is that you can find just about any exercise you desire.

One of the fun things about apps and videos is that you don't have to leave the comfort of your home (yes, it's possible to do leg lifts in your pajamas). You don't have to be embarrassed about how you look in workout gear or that you don't know the steps or that you sweat a lot. Maybe you need to take a lot of breaks. No problem. Just pause it.

Apps can also keep track of your activity and help you set and reach goals. And that can be fun, too. You can do this on your own or participate with a group of friends to get alerts on one another's progress and encourage one another to keep moving.

TIP

YouTube, iTunes, and Google Play are flooded with terrific exercise videos and apps. Look for highly rated ones with lots of views or subscribers. You'll have to pay for some, but there are excellent free apps and videos, too.

Turn Up the Volume

Whether you prefer a Beyoncé dance track or Tchaikovsky's *Swan Lake*, music can make your workout more fun. Why? Music makes us want to move, whether it's the beat or the emotions it evokes. We can't help it.

Music can also be distracting, in a good way. Just when you're tired and sweaty and don't think you could take another step, your favorite song comes on and — *voilà!* — you're swept away to the beat. You're no longer thinking about stopping, you're thinking about how Taylor Swift is telling you to "Shake It Off."

TECHNICAL
STUFF

In a small study from 2017, researchers found that people who exercised to music were more positive about their interval-training exercises than people who exercised without music.

Think Positive

Have you heard about the power of positive thoughts? Well, it certainly sounds like a good thing. And research shows that positive thinking can have health benefits, too. For example, a 2013 study showed that people with a family history of heart disease who also had a positive outlook were one-third less likely to have coronary artery disease than those with a negative outlook.

The next time you're thinking that exercise is decidedly un-fun, try shifting your brain. Instead, think about exercise as a wonderful opportunity. Think about how great it is that you can still exercise.

REMEMBER

Some positive thoughts about your own body won't hurt either. The next time you hear yourself thinking that you're out of shape, you're overweight, or you can't do this, turn the conversation around. Instead, tell yourself you're doing good things to take care of your body. Tell yourself that your body is strong and capable. It's much more fun to be good to yourself than it is to knock yourself down.

Volunteer to Help Someone Else

The next time you're feeling down about exercise, consider volunteering. Helping other people is, well, helpful of course, but it also has health benefits. A 2013 review of studies in the journal *BMC Public Health* found that volunteering had favorable benefits on mental health such as satisfaction, well-being, and depression, although not specifically physical health.

Volunteer for something that gets you moving, like delivering food to people through Meals on Wheels or working at a local soup kitchen or maintaining hiking or biking trails in your community. If you really want to get moving, volunteer for Habitat for Humanity to build houses for underserved communities. Go to Volunteers of America (www.voa.org) to find opportunities in your neighborhood.

Sign Up for a Walk to Raise Money

Walking for a cause like raising funds for diabetes, heart disease, or cancer research can be fun and rewarding. For one thing, you'll have an event that might motivate you to get in shape or just start walking more regularly. This might be just the incentive you need to start walking at lunch or on the weekends.

You'll also meet people at the event who share your interests and motivations. For example, if you have type 2 diabetes, you'll meet a lot of people at an American Diabetes Association walk who struggle with the same issues as you. You might also break the sense of isolation that comes with having a chronic condition or taking care of someone with a chronic condition. It's easy to feel alone, so take the opportunity to meet other people, raise some money (or just awareness), and get some exercise to boot.

Set Realistic and Practical Goals

Setting realistic and practical goals probably doesn't sound like much fun. But there's a silver lining to this approach: You're more likely to exercise and lose weight if you set goals that are small and that you can achieve. And there's nothing more exciting than stepping on that scale and seeing you dropped 1 or 2 pounds!

What's a realistic and practical goal? Well, it depends on your age, your current physical activity, your lifestyle and work schedule, and many other things.

However, it's a given that just saying you're going to lose 15 pounds isn't going to make it happen. That goal is too vague and far away to be feasible.

Instead, you'll need to make a plan for achieving a weight loss goal, of say 5 pounds (or another small increment) by coming up with daily, weekly, and even monthly strategies. Your plan might include scheduling specific exercise and workouts ahead of time. You might need to work with a personal trainer or diabetes educator to define your goals and track your progress. Setting and achieving smaller, realistic goals can help keep you motivated and moving forward.

Just Dance

Dancing could be one of the most under-appreciated ways to burn calories. The next time you're feeling bored out of your gourd by the thought of exercise, turn on some music and have a dance party.

You could invite your kids or spouse, but don't be shy about breaking out your best moves on your own (just like Tom Cruise in *Risky Business*). You don't need the white socks, but "Old Time Rock & Roll" by Bob Seger is never a bad music choice.

Or you may be more moved by a dance that evokes your culture and traditions. Sign up for a dance class at a cultural or community center, or dance to a YouTube video in the privacy of your own room. Turning on music while you cook dinner might inspire you to shake your hips and take a few extra steps as you're sautéing vegetables at the stove.

Chapter **21**

Ten (Or So) Things to Do for Your Eyes

Your eyes and eyesight are precious resources, and you need to take extra steps to preserve them when you have type 2 diabetes. It can be easy to take your vision for granted. It's one of those senses that most of us rely on almost 24/7, unless we're sleeping of course. And even then, we might need our peepers to help us find the bathroom light in the middle of the night.

Some say that eyes are the windows to the soul. For people with diabetes, the eyes are certainly the windows into your health. Your eyes can be protected or damaged by your blood glucose control, and they're often a microcosm of your greater diabetes care. Turn to Chapter 8 for more information on how the eye works. Read on for tips on keeping your eyes healthy for years to come.

Keep Your Blood Glucose in Control

You'll need to keep your blood glucose on target to keep your eyes healthy. Why would blood glucose matter at all to your eyes? Well, your retina contains those all-important specialized cells (rods and cones) that help you see clearly. Blood vessels supply the retina with necessary blood and nutrients to keep those cells in tip-top condition. Blood vessels also supply nerves in your eyes.

High blood glucose damages blood vessels and nerves by slowing or lessening the flow of blood. When this happens, the cells in your retina are, in a way, starved of what they need to survive and flourish, leading to eye disease called *diabetic retinopathy* (described in more detail later in this chapter). High blood glucose can increase your risk for cataracts and nerve damage in your eye.

In the short term, high blood glucose can also lead to blurry vision, a symptom that can prompt a person to see a doctor and lead to a diagnosis of diabetes. Sometimes this might happen if you're experiencing hyperglycemia (an episode of high blood glucose) or if you're changing medications. Likely, the blurry vision will go away once your blood glucose returns to normal.

REMEMBER

The American Diabetes Association recommends a reasonable goal for many with diabetes of A1C below 7 percent, as well as a fasting blood glucose of 80–130 mg/dL and a blood glucose of less than 180 mg/dL 1–2 hours after meals. Ask your diabetes care provider about your ideal blood glucose and A1C targets.

Lower Your Blood Pressure and Cholesterol

Lowering your blood pressure and cholesterol will help keep the blood vessels in your eyes healthy. High blood pressure and high cholesterol damage blood vessels and nerves by blocking the supply of essential blood and nutrients. Much like high blood glucose, these things can lead to diabetic retinopathy, optic neuropathy, and buildup of fluid in the retina.

REMEMBER

Your diabetes care team should measure your blood pressure at every checkup. The American Diabetes Association recommends less than 140 mm/Hg systolic blood pressure and less than 90 mm/Hg diastolic blood pressure.

TIP

To lower your blood pressure, eat wholesome, nutritious foods that are low in sodium. Exercise regularly and try to lose weight. You may need to take medication, such as ACE inhibitors, angiotensin II receptor blockers (ARBs), and other drugs, to lower your blood pressure.

You should also have your blood lipids (cholesterol and other blood fats) measured at diagnosis and every 5 years after, or as needed. Your diabetes care provider may prescribe medication to lower your bad cholesterol, and you should exercise, eat healthy foods, and lose weight if possible.

Stop Smoking or Never Start

Everyone knows that smoking is bad for your health. But did you know smoking can also lead to vision impairment and eye disease? Yep, add your eyesight to the long list of reasons to quit smoking (or never start).

Smoking raises your blood pressure, which, as explained in the preceding section, can damage the blood vessels in your eyes. People who smoke have a greater risk for two eye diseases, macular degeneration and cataracts, which can both lead to vision loss including blindness. People with diabetes are at greater risk for glaucoma, cataracts, and other eye diseases, so quitting smoking is a must.

TIP

Call 800-QUIT-NOW or visit www.smokefree.gov for resources on quitting smoking.

Be Aware of Major Eye Diseases

Diabetic retinopathy is the number one cause of blindness among working-age adults in the United States. It's caused by high blood glucose and leads to several changes in your eyeballs. There are two types of diabetic retinopathy:

>> **Background retinopathy:** In background retinopathy, tiny blood vessels (called *capillaries*) rupture and spill blood and fluid. This can lead to scarring and loss of vision. The reduced blood flow can also damage nerve tissue. It can cause *diabetic macular edema* (DME), swelling of the retina's macula area that can impair central vision (used for driving, reading, and so on). Injections and laser surgery can be effective treatments (see more about them later in this chapter).

>> **Proliferative retinopathy:** In the more serious proliferative neuropathy, reduced blood flow prompts your body to make more small blood vessels in your eyes. That's how it gets its name; *proliferative* means to grow rapidly. However, these new blood vessels are fragile and rupture easily, sometimes leading to a sudden loss of vision or scarring that can lead to a detached retina.

Glaucoma is an eye disease in which high blood pressure damages the optic nerve, which can lead to vision impairment. People with diabetes are more likely to have glaucoma than people without diabetes. Lowering your blood pressure will decrease your risk for this eye disease.

Cataracts are cloudy parts of your lens, which can blur your vision. High blood glucose can cause your lenses to swell and become cloudy, both of which increase your risk for cataracts. People with diabetes are more likely to have cataracts than people without diabetes.

REMEMBER

High blood glucose and high blood pressure put your whole body at risk, so if you find out you have eye disease, ask about other potential complications. For example, people with diabetes and severe retinopathy are twice as likely to have coronary heart disease than people without retinopathy. And they have a three times higher risk of it being deadly. People with diabetes and eye disease are also more likely to have kidney disease. (And the opposite is true: People with kidney disease due to diabetes have a very high likelihood of having eye disease as well.)

Get Regular Dilated Eye Exams

A dilated eye exam is the best way to detect and prevent the progression of diabetic eye diseases — and help preserve your vision for years to come. It's truly your most powerful weapon to keep your eyesight. Many of the eye diseases mentioned in the preceding section can be treated effectively when caught early enough. However, the only way to catch these eye diseases is with a dilated eye exam.

Why is a dilated eye exam necessary? You may not notice vision damage before it's too late. Sometimes there are no warning signs. Yet, an ophthalmologist or optometrist employs specialized tools to look inside your eye — all the way to your retina and optic nerve — to detect changes.

REMEMBER

The American Diabetes Association recommends that every person with type 2 diabetes receive a dilated eye exam at diagnosis. Then you should have an eye exam every 1–2 years after, depending on your provider's recommendation.

In a dilated eye exam, your eye-care provider will dilate your eyes using drops. The drops make your retina big — really big — and allow more light into the back of your eye. This allows your provider to see your whole retina, macula, and optic nerve. She'll use a special magnifying glass to inspect the blood vessels and other important parts.

Tonometry is a fancy name for measuring the pressure in your eye, and it's used to detect glaucoma. Your eye-care provider will check your *peripheral* (or side) *vision* for signs of damage. You'll also get a vision test to check whether you can see clearly up close or at a distance. This is that black-and-white eye chart with the giant E at the tippy top. You can then be measured for glasses or contact lenses if needed.

Get the Treatment You Need

Blindness (see the "Be Aware of Major Eye Diseases" section earlier in this chapter) can be reduced by 90 percent if diabetic retinopathy is caught early and treated. That's an amazing number. Injections and laser surgery can treat diabetic retinopathy. For example, anti-VEGF injections can treat diabetic macular edema. Also, a surgical procedure can improve retinal detachment. Cataracts can be treated by replacing the damaged lens with an artificial lens to restore vision. Eye drops can help treat glaucoma, and laser and other types of surgery can be used, too.

If your optometrist or ophthalmologist diagnoses eye disease, make sure you schedule treatment even if you don't feel like there's anything wrong. You may not have any symptoms or vision problems — and yet you may still need treatment to preserve your vision.

REMEMBER

The ACCORD study showed that intensive glucose control can reduce the risk of progression of diabetic retinopathy in people with type 2 diabetes. Keeping your blood glucose on target really does help!

Consider Your Eyes during Pregnancy

You're focused on the baby growing inside you when you become pregnant — and rightly so. If you had type 2 diabetes before you became pregnant, your diabetes care team is probably working with you to make sure you manage your blood glucose during pregnancy. You're probably watching what you eat and monitoring your blood glucose more closely. Another thing to keep in mind: your eyes.

Diabetic retinopathy can develop and progress rapidly during pregnancy for women with preexisting type 2 diabetes. Sometimes this coincides with the more intensive blood glucose management that is recommended during pregnancy.

REMEMBER

If you have type 2 diabetes, the American Diabetes Association recommends a dilated exam before you become pregnant or during your first trimester. Then have an eye exam during each trimester and the year following your baby's birth.

Assess Your Risk Factors

Hispanic Americans are more likely to have diabetic retinopathy than people of other races. Also, a family history of glaucoma is a risk factor for this type of eye disease.

Adolescents with type 2 diabetes are more likely to develop retinopathy than adolescents with type 1 diabetes — and perhaps with more severity. One study found that most kids with type 2 diabetes don't get eye exams despite health insurance coverage, even within 6 years of diagnosis.

The number of Americans with diabetic retinopathy is expected to double from 2010 to 2050, going from 7.7 million to 14.6 million, according to the National Institutes of Health's National Eye Institute.

Glossary

acesulfame-K: *See* acesulfame potassium.

acesulfame potassium: A sweetener with no calories and no nutritional value. Brand names: Sunett, Sweet One. *Also known as* acesulfame-K.

acute: Sudden and lasting for a short time; often accompanied by a sharp rise in severity. *See also* chronic.

Adequate Intake (AI): One of the four reference values for the Dietary Reference Intake (DRI) based on observed or experimentally determined estimates of nutrient intake by a group of healthy people. These nutrients are assumed to be adequate. Used when a Recommended Dietary Allowance (RDA) cannot be determined.

adipose tissue: A connective tissue that stores fat for energy, insulation, and cushioning. Adipose tissue, especially within the abdomen, produces hormones and substances that cause inflammation; these factors can contribute to insulin resistance and type 2 diabetes. Prevention of type 2 diabetes is linked to controlling or reducing excess body weight. Commonly referred to as *fat*.

adult-onset diabetes: *See* type 2 diabetes.

Advantame: An artificial sweetener with few calories and no nutritional value. It is 20,000 times sweeter than table sugar.

aerobic exercise: Rapid physical activity that works the heart, lungs, arms, legs, and the rest of the body; typically causes harder breathing and faster heart rate.

Affordable Care Act: A law that reformed health insurance to make it more affordable, more accessible, and of higher quality. A marketplace was created for comparison of health plans. Tax credits are available to middle- and low-income families to help pay for insurance premiums. Under this law, a consumer with a preexisting condition can no longer be denied insurance. *Also known as* Obamacare.

a-glucosidase inhibitor: *See* alpha-glucosidase inhibitor.

albiglutide: An injectable glucagon-like peptide-1 (GLP-1) agonist. Used for improving glycemic control in adults with type 2 diabetes. Brand name: Tanzeum.

albumin: A protein found in animal tissues, manufactured by the liver and circulated in human blood. Increased amounts in the urine can be a sign of early diabetic kidney damage.

albumin excretion rate (AER): A urine test that measures the amount of albumin in the urine to determine kidney health.

albuminuria: A condition in which the urine has more than normal amounts of albumin; often an early sign of diabetic nephropathy (kidney disease).

alogliptin: An oral hypoglycemic agent used to treat type 2 diabetes. It belongs to the class of medications called dipeptidyl peptidase-4 inhibitors. Brand name: Nesina.

alpha-glucosidase inhibitor: A class of oral medicine for type 2 diabetes that blocks the enzymes that digest starches in food. The result is a slower and lower rise in blood glucose after meals. Generic names: acarbose, miglitol. *Also known as* a-glucosidase inhibitor.

Americans with Disabilities Act: An act signed into law in 1990 that prohibits discrimination against people with disabilities, especially with regard to employment and government programs. A *disability* is defined as a physical or mental impairment that substantially limits one or more of a person's major life activities.

amylin: A hormone formed by beta cells in the pancreas; regulates the timing of glucose release into the bloodstream after eating by slowing the emptying of the stomach.

analog: An organic compound that has a structure and function similar to another organic compound. Examples include insulin analog, amylin analog, and GLP-1 analog.

angiopathy: Any disease of the blood vessels (veins, arteries, and capillaries).

angiotensin: A substance in the blood that constricts the blood vessels and thereby increases blood pressure.

angiotensin receptor blocker (ARB): An oral medicine that is used to treat hypertension.

antihypertensive drug: Any of a class of medications that lowers blood pressure to treat hypertension, including ACE inhibitors, beta blockers, ARBs, calcium antagonists, calcium channel blockers, and thiazide diuretics.

antioxidant: A chemical substance that helps protect against cell damage caused by free radicals. Examples include vitamin A, vitamin C, and vitamin E.

A1C test: A test that shows a person's average blood glucose level over the past 2–3 months, usually shown as a percentage. The A1C test measures the amount of glycated hemoglobin (also called hemoglobin A1C, or HbA1c) in the blood. Often reported along with estimated average glucose (eAG).

aspartame: A low-calorie sweetener with almost no calories and almost no nutritional value. Brand names: Equal, NutraSweet, Sugar Twin.

aspart insulin: A rapid-acting insulin that, on average, starts to lower blood glucose levels within 10–20 minutes after injection, has its strongest effect 30–60 minutes after injection, and keeps working for 3–5 hours after injection. Brand name: Novolog.

autonomic neuropathy: A disease that affects part of the nervous system not under conscious control. It may cause slowed emptying of the stomach, difficulty regulating blood pressure, and other complications.

background diabetic retinopathy: A type of damage to the retina of the eye marked by small hemorrhages and abnormal dilation of the blood vessels; usually causes no symptoms; an early stage of diabetic retinopathy. *Also known as* non-proliferative retinopathy.

bariatrics: The branch of medicine that deals with the causes, prevention, and treatment of obesity.

bariatric surgery: A surgical procedure for weight loss that restricts the amount of food that goes into the stomach with or without preventing the body from fully digesting all the nutrients from the food that is eaten. Examples include gastric bypass, adjustable gastric band, and sleeve gastrectomy.

basal insulin: (1) An intermediate- or long-acting insulin that is absorbed slowly and gives the body a steady, low level of insulin to manage blood glucose levels between meals, thus mimicking the body's natural, low-level, steady background release of insulin; background insulin. (2) The low-level, steady background release of insulin by an insulin pump.

behavioral therapy: An approach to treatment in which specific behaviors are targeted for change, including the ideas and emotions associated with that behavior; often used to adjust eating habits to encourage weight loss.

beta blocker: An antihypertensive drug.

beta cell: A cell that makes insulin and amylin and is located in the islet cells of the pancreas. Also written as β-cell.

biguanide: A class of oral medicine used to treat type 2 diabetes; lowers blood glucose by reducing the amount of glucose produced by the liver and by helping the body respond better to insulin. Generic name: metformin.

blood fat: A lipid (or fat) carried through the blood by a lipoprotein; usually used to refer to cholesterol and triglycerides.

blood glucose (BG): The main sugar found in the blood and the body's main energy source. *Also known as* blood sugar.

blood glucose meter: A small, portable machine used by people with diabetes to check their blood glucose levels. After pricking the skin with a lancet, you place a drop of blood on a test strip in the machine, and then the meter (or monitor) displays the blood glucose level on a digital display.

blood glucose monitoring: The process and procedure of checking blood glucose levels to manage diabetes, usually with the aid of a blood glucose meter.

blood sugar: *See* blood glucose (BG).

body mass index (BMI): A method of evaluating the body's weight relative to its height and represented as weight in kilograms divided by the square of the height in meters (kg/m^2); used to determine the following categories: underweight, normal weight, overweight, or obese. This measurement correlates highly with body fat.

bolus insulin: An extra amount of insulin taken to cover an expected rise in blood glucose, often related to a meal or snack.

bromocriptine: An oral medicine used to regulate blood glucose levels in patients with type 2 diabetes. Brand name: Cycloset.

calcium antagonist: *See* calcium channel blocker (CCB).

calcium channel blocker (CCB): A class of antihypertensive drug. *Also known as* calcium antagonist.

carbohydrate (CHO, carb): One of the three primary nutrients found in food, primarily in starches, vegetables, fruits, dairy products, and sugars.

carbohydrate counting: A method of meal planning for people with diabetes based on counting the number of grams of carbohydrate in the food that is to be consumed.

cardiometabolic risk factors: A set of risk factors that, when viewed together, are good indicators of a person's overall risk of developing heart disease and type 2 diabetes. These risk factors include obesity, high LDL cholesterol, high triglycerides, low HDL cholesterol, hypertension, smoking, and physical inactivity. Each of these risk factors poses a danger to good health, and the more one has, the greater the risk of heart disease and type 2 diabetes.

cardiovascular disease (CVD): *See* macrovascular disease (MVD).

casual plasma glucose test: *See* random plasma glucose test.

celiac disease: A condition in which gluten causes an autoimmune attack that damages the intestines, an organ that helps digest food; therefore, nutrients are not absorbed properly, which can lead to many other complications. Celiac disease arises more frequently in people with type 1 diabetes and is generally treated by prescribing a gluten-free diet. *Also known as* celiac sprue, gluten-sensitive enteropathy, *or* nontropical sprue.

celiac sprue: *See* celiac disease.

certified diabetes educator (CDE): A healthcare professional with expertise in diabetes education and who has met eligibility requirements and successfully completed a certification exam.

chronic: Long lasting. *See also* acute.

co-insurance: A co-payment for fee-for-service health plans, usually represented as a percentage of cost (for example, the insurance company pays 75 percent of the claim, and the insured pays the remaining 25 percent).

combination medication: Two or more active medications combined into a single dose form. Examples include metaglip, a combination of metformin and glipizide.

combination therapy: The use of different medicines together, such as multiple oral medications or one or more oral medications and insulin, to manage the blood glucose levels in people with type 2 diabetes.

complex carbohydrate: *See* starch.

complication: A harmful condition that results from the effects of diabetes on the body, such as damage to the eyes, heart, blood vessels, nervous system, teeth, gums, feet, skin, and kidneys.

Consolidated Omnibus Budget Reconciliation Act (COBRA): A federal law enacted in 1986. Under this act, an employer with more than 20 employees must allow a former employee and his or her dependents to retain the same health insurance policy with equal coverage for 18–36 months after leaving the job. The former employee has to pay for the coverage and may be charged up to 2 percent. The insurance can be used until coverage is found through the Affordable Care Act marketplace.

continuous glucose monitor (CGM): A device that continuously records glucose levels throughout the day and night through a subcutaneously implanted sensor. The measurement is done on fluid between cells (interstitial fluid), and the levels are very similar to blood glucose levels. The system is used to measure glucose levels to help identify fluctuations and trends that would otherwise go unnoticed with standard A1C tests and finger-stick measurements.

continuous subcutaneous insulin infusion (CSII): The method by which insulin pumps deliver insulin. A steady, measured amount of basal insulin is delivered under the skin (subcutaneously).

contraindication: A condition or situation that increases the risks involved in using a particular drug, carrying out a medical procedure, or engaging in a particular activity, thus making the treatment inadvisable.

co-payment: A method of sharing costs between an insurance company and its members; often a discounted flat fee is paid every time the member receives a medical service.

coronary artery disease (CAD): *See* coronary heart disease (CHD).

coronary heart disease (CHD): A condition caused by narrowing of the arteries that supply blood to the heart; can result in a myocardial infarction. *Also known as* coronary artery disease (CAD).

counterregulatory hormone: A hormone released during stressful situations or in response to hypoglycemia, including glucagon, epinephrine (adrenaline), norepinephrine, cortisol, and growth hormone. Such hormones tell the liver to release glucose and the fat cells to release fatty acids for extra energy. If the body does not have enough insulin present when these hormones are released, hyperglycemia and diabetic ketoacidosis can result.

C-peptide: The abbreviation for *connecting peptide,* a substance released by the beta cells into the bloodstream in amounts equal to those of insulin; testing levels of C-peptide reveals how much insulin the body is making.

dawn phenomenon: The early-morning (4–8 a.m.) rise in blood glucose level due to hormones.

deductible: A set amount of money that a person must pay each year to cover medical care expenses before the insurance company begins paying.

dermatologist: A doctor who specializes in diagnosing and treating problems of the skin and hair.

detemir insulin: A long-acting insulin analog used to provide a basal or background insulin level. Brand name: Levemir.

dextrose: *See* glucose.

diabetes burnout: A condition that may affect people with diabetes in which the burdens and constant requirements of diabetes self-management eventually cause the patient to become overwhelmed and frustrated, resulting in lost motivation. People suffering from diabetes burnout often feel defeated by diabetes or angry about having diabetes, and try to avoid or cease diabetes care.

diabetes education and support: A program or general curriculum that aims to teach people with diabetes how to address and care for the daily demands of diabetes. Diabetes self-management support is an ongoing process that encourages behavior change and addresses psychosocial concerns. Diabetes education courses and programs usually cover the following topics: general information about diabetes and its treatments, psychological adjustments to life with diabetes, setting goals and solving problems, setting and following a meal plan, increasing exercise, blood glucose monitoring, managing sick days, and identifying and preventing complications.

Diabetes Medical Management Plan: An individualized care plan for children to be used at school. The plan is created by the child's diabetes care provider, and parents or guardians are responsible for giving the plan to the child's school. Each plan is different, because there are different ways to treat or monitor blood glucose levels, and each individual needs different levels of support.

diabetes mellitus: A condition characterized by hyperglycemia resulting from the body's inability to use blood glucose for energy. In type 1 diabetes, the pancreas no longer makes insulin; therefore, blood glucose cannot enter the cells to be used for energy. In type 2 diabetes, the pancreas does not make enough insulin, and the body is unable to use insulin correctly.

diabetic ketoacidosis (DKA): An emergency condition in which extreme hyperglycemia, along with a severe lack of insulin, results in the breakdown of body fat for energy and an accumulation of ketones in the blood and urine. Signs are nausea, vomiting, stomach pain, fruity odor on the breath, and rapid breathing. If left untreated, it can lead to coma and death.

diabetic neuropathy (DN): Nerve damage that arises as a complication of diabetes.

diabetic retinopathy: Damage to the small blood vessels in the retina that arises as a complication of diabetes. If untreated, loss of vision can result.

diabetologist: A doctor who specializes in treating people with diabetes.

dietary fiber: The fiber contained in the diet, consisting of both soluble and insoluble fiber. General recommendations are 25–30 grams of fiber per day.

Dietary Reference Intake (DRI): The compilation of several indexes of dietary intake that can be used to evaluate or plan diets for individuals and groups. The four main reference values that comprise the Dietary Reference Intake are Recommended Dietary Allowance, Adequate Intake, Tolerable Upper Intake Level, and Estimated Average Requirement. There are dietary reference intakes for vitamins, elements, macronutrients, electrolytes, and water, as well as the recommended intakes for individuals.

dietitian: A healthcare professional who advises people about meal planning, weight control, and diabetes management. A registered dietitian (RD) has more training.

dilated eye exam: A test done by an eye-care specialist in which the *pupil* (the black center) of the eye is temporarily enlarged with eye drops to allow the specialist to more easily see the inside of the eye.

dipeptidyl peptidase-4 inhibitor: A class of oral hypoglycemic agents that block the action of dipeptidyl peptidase-4. By blocking the action of dipeptidyl peptidase-4, the action of glucagon-like peptide-1 is prolonged, allowing the secretion of more insulin to counteract high blood glucose levels. Examples include vildagliptin and sitagliptin.

distal symmetric polyneuropathy: *See* peripheral neuropathy.

d-phenylalanine derivative: A class of oral medicine for type 2 diabetes that lowers blood glucose levels by helping the pancreas make more insulin right after meals. Generic name: nateglinide.

dyslipidemia: Abnormal blood fat levels, usually referring to high levels of LDL cholesterol, low levels of HDL cholesterol, and/or high levels of triglycerides.

endocrinologist: A doctor who treats people who have endocrine gland problems, such as diabetes.

endocrinology: The study of diseases related to hormones produced by the body.

end-stage renal disease: *See* kidney failure.

epidemiology: The study of disease patterns in populations of humans that deals with how many people have that particular disease, where the population is located, how many new cases of the disease develop, and how the disease is controlled.

erectile dysfunction (ED): The inability to get or maintain an erection; a complication of diabetes that can often be treated with medication. *Also known as* impotence.

estimated average glucose (eAG): A numerical value calculated from the A1C that shows a person's average blood glucose levels over a period of 2–3 months; reported in the same units as real-time blood glucose levels taken with a blood glucose meter, milligrams per deciliter (mg/dL). Estimated average glucose was developed to give people with diabetes more meaningful information beyond A1C, which is reported in percentages in the United States and in mmol/mol in some other countries.

Estimated Average Requirement (EAR): One of the four reference values of the Dietary Reference Intake; estimates the amount of a nutrient needed to meet the requirement of half of the healthy individuals in an age-group and gender group; used to assess dietary adequacy and as the basis for the Recommended Dietary Allowance.

estimated glomerular filtration rate (eGER): A test that evaluates kidney function and checks for kidney damage. The results from this test are estimated from the results of a creatinine test, which is part of the routine set of lab tests called a *metabolic panel.*

exclusive provider organization (EPO): A type of managed-care organization; specifically, a type of preferred provider organization in which individual members use assigned physicians instead of having a choice of a variety of providers.

exenatide: A glucagon-like peptide-1 (GLP-1) agonist that is injected; used to improve blood glucose control in adults with type 2 diabetes. Brand name: Byetta.

exercise physiologist: A specialist trained in the science of exercise and body conditioning who can help patients plan a safe, effective exercise program.

fasting blood glucose (FBG) test: *See* fasting plasma glucose (FPG) test.

fasting plasma glucose (FPG) test: A test that checks a person's blood glucose level after the person has not eaten for 8–12 hours (usually overnight); used to diagnose prediabetes and diabetes and to monitor blood glucose levels in people with diabetes. If blood glucose levels are above normal but not high enough to diagnose diabetes, this is termed *impaired fasting glucose. Also known as* fasting blood glucose (FBG) test.

fat: (1) One of the main nutrients in food. Foods that provide fat include butter, margarine, salad dressing, oil, nuts, meat, poultry, fish, and some dairy products. (2) Any of the different kinds of fat found in food, including monounsaturated fat, omega-3 fatty acid, polyunsaturated fat, saturated fat, and trans fatty acid. (3) Excess calories stored as adipose tissue (also called body fat), which provides the body with a reserve supply of energy, keeps it insulated, and cushions it. (4) When in the body, particularly in the bloodstream, often called a *lipid* or *blood fat.*

fee-for-service healthcare: A type of healthcare insurance in which the insurance company pays for the services and costs incurred by the insured person. The insured person has the flexibility to select the hospital, clinic, and/or doctors; however, the insurance company will often not pay 100 percent of the medical expenses incurred. People belonging to such a plan can expect to pay a monthly fee (or premium), a deductible, and, if applicable, co-insurance.

15-gram/15-minute rule: A method of treating hypoglycemia; when blood glucose levels are low, the patient takes a 15-gram carbohydrate source (such as a glucose tablet, ½ cup juice, or 1 cup nonfat milk), waits 15 minutes, and then checks levels again. If blood glucose levels remain low, the patient repeats the process until the levels optimize. *Also known as* Rule of 15.

50/50 insulin: Premixed insulin that is 50 percent intermediate-acting insulin and 50 percent short-acting (regular) insulin.

504 Plan: A plan developed to meet the requirements of a federal law that prohibits discrimination against people with disabilities, Section 504 of the Rehabilitation Act of 1973. Section 504 applies to all public schools and to private schools that receive federal funds. A 504 Plan sets out an agreement to ensure that the student has the same access to education as other children. It is used to make sure the student, the parents/guardians, and school personnel understand their responsibilities and to prepare for possible problem situations.

flexibility exercise: Any of the many physical activities that increase the body's flexibility. *Also known as* stretching.

focal neuropathy: A condition due to damage to a single nerve or group of nerves that usually goes away in 2 weeks to 18 months; caused either by blockage of a blood vessel that supplies the nerve or nerves with blood or by a pinched nerve. Examples include carpal tunnel syndrome.

food choices: A method of diabetes meal planning. Foods are categorized into seven groups based on nutritional content and a standardized serving size: starch, protein, vegetables, fruits, milk and milk substitutes, fat, and other carbohydrates. This was formerly known as the exchange list system of meal planning.

fructosamine test: A measure of the number of blood glucose molecules linked to protein molecules in the blood; provides information on average blood glucose levels for the past 2–3 weeks; often used in patients who cannot undergo the A1C test (for example, a person with anemia).

fructose: A sugar that occurs naturally in fruits and honey; has 4 calories per gram.

gastric bypass surgery: A bariatric surgical procedure in which the stomach is made smaller and digestion bypasses part of the small intestine; often done to help patients lose large amounts of body weight, particularly those with a body mass index over 35 kg/m².

gastroparesis: A form of neuropathy that affects the stomach. Digestion of food may be incomplete or delayed, resulting in nausea, vomiting, or bloating, making blood glucose levels difficult to control.

gestational diabetes mellitus (GDM): A type of diabetes that develops only during pregnancy and usually disappears upon delivery, but increases the risk that the mother will later develop diabetes; managed with meal planning, physical activity, and sometimes insulin.

glargine insulin: A long-acting basal insulin analog that, on average, starts to lower blood glucose levels within 1 hour after injection and keeps working relatively evenly for about 24 hours after injection. Brand name: Lantus.

glimepiride: An oral medicine used to treat type 2 diabetes and belonging to the class of medicines called sulfonylureas. Brand name: Amaryl.

glipizide: An oral medicine used to treat type 2 diabetes and belonging to the class of medicines called sulfonylureas. Brand names: Glucotrol, Glucotrol XL.

glomerular filtration rate: A measure of the ability of the kidneys to filter and remove waste products.

glucagon: A hormone produced by the alpha cells in the pancreas that raises blood glucose levels. An injectable form of glucagon, available by prescription, may be used to treat severe hypoglycemia.

glucagon-like peptide-1 (GLP-1): An incretin that increases insulin secretion from the pancreas. Medicines that mimic this peptide can be helpful in treating diabetes.

glucometer: *See* blood glucose meter.

glucose: One of the simplest forms of carbohydrate; a simple sugar found in blood that serves as the body's main source of energy. It can also be ingested to treat hypoglycemia (for example, glucose tablets or gel). *Also known as* dextrose.

glucose metabolism: The process by which glucose is converted to energy.

glucose tablet: A chewable tablet made of pure glucose; used to treat hypoglycemia.

glulisine insulin: A rapid-acting insulin analog. On average, glulisine insulin starts to lower blood glucose levels within 15 minutes after injection. It has its strongest effect 1–1½ hours after injection and keeps working for about 3 hours after injection. Brand name: Apidra.

gluten: A type of protein found in wheat, rye, barley, and some other grains, including most common flours; can also be found in certain medications and in some store-bought items (for example, some brands of soy sauce).

gluten-free diet: The prescribed treatment for celiac disease, in which a person has no gluten in his or her daily diet.

gluten-sensitive enteropathy: *See* celiac disease.

glyburide: An oral medicine used to treat type 2 diabetes and belonging to the class of medicines called sulfonylureas. Brand names: DiaBeta, Glynase PresTab, Micronase.

glycated hemoglobin (GHb, HbA1c): A form of hemoglobin to which glucose has joined; in people with diabetes, the amount of glycated hemoglobin is increased and can be measured to determine average blood glucose levels over a certain period of time (*see* A1C test). Often it is co-reported with eAG. *Also known as* glycohemoglobin *and* hemoglobin A1c.

glycemic index: A ranking of carbohydrate-containing foods, based on the food's effect on blood glucose levels compared with a standard reference food.

glycemic load: A measurement of the impact that the carbohydrate in a certain food will have on blood glucose levels. It's calculated by multiplying a food's glycemic index by its amount of carbohydrate. Food items are designated as having a low, medium, or high glycemic load.

glycogen: The form of stored glucose found in the liver and muscles.

glycohemoglobin: *See* glycated hemoglobin (GHb, HbA1c).

glycosuria: The presence of glucose in the urine.

group insurance: A health insurance policy issued by an employer in which groups of employees (and sometimes dependents) are covered under a single policy or contract.

HbA1c: *See* glycated hemoglobin (GHb, HbA1c).

healthcare team: A group of healthcare professionals who work with a patient to help in the care of a chronic disease (a process called *team management*); often used in the treatment of diabetes and may include a primary-care doctor, diabetes educator, dietitian, exercise physiologist, optometrist, podiatrist, and pharmacist.

Health Insurance Portability and Accountability Act (HIPPA): A law enacted in 1996 under which insurers and employers may not make insurance rules that discriminate against workers because of their health. All workers eligible for a certain health insurance plan must be offered enrollment at the same price. The law also covers the protection of personal medical information in multiple ways and establishes a national standard for electronic security that all businesses must use.

health maintenance organization (HMO): A type of managed care organization that is a prepaid health insurance plan; members pay a monthly premium for comprehensive care from the organization's hospitals, offices, and staff, which are only available to members.

heart disease: A condition that affects the heart muscle, heart valves, or the blood vessels of the heart.

hemoglobin: The protein in a red blood cell that carries oxygen to the cells.

hemoglobin A1c: *See* glycated hemoglobin (GHb, HbA1c).

high blood pressure: *See* hypertension (HTN).

high-density lipoprotein (HDL) cholesterol: A fat found in the blood in a particle that takes extra cholesterol to the liver for removal; often called *good cholesterol* or *healthy cholesterol.*

honeymoon phase: A temporary remission of type 1 diabetes that sometimes occurs soon after the diagnosis of diabetes is made. During this time, the pancreas may still secrete some insulin, but over time, this secretion will stop. This condition can last weeks, months, or a year or longer.

hyperglycemia: Excessively high blood glucose levels; signs include excessive thirst (polydipsia), excessive urination (polyuria), and excessive hunger (polyphagia), but more moderate levels of hyperglycemia often cause no symptoms.

hyperinsulinemia: A condition in which the level of insulin in the blood is higher than normal; caused by overproduction of insulin by the body; related to insulin resistance.

hyperlipidemia: Higher-than-normal triglyceride or cholesterol levels in the blood.

hypernatremia: A condition characterized by excessive amounts of sodium in the blood, usually due to a lack of fluid in the body; can be an indicator of diabetes insipidus.

hyperosmolar hyperglycemic nonketotic syndrome (HHNS): *See* hyperosmolar hyperglycemic syndrome (HHS).

hyperosmolar hyperglycemic syndrome (HHS): An emergency condition in which a person's blood glucose level is very high, but ketones are not present in the blood or urine. If left untreated, it can lead to coma or death. *Also known as* hyperosmolar hyperglycemic nonketotic syndrome (HHNS).

hypertension (HTN): A condition present when blood flows through the blood vessels with a force greater than normal, potentially straining the heart, damaging blood vessels, and increasing the risk of heart attack, stroke, and kidney disease. *Also known as* high blood pressure.

hypoglycemia: A condition characterized by abnormally low blood glucose levels, usually less than 70 mg/dL; signs include hunger, nervousness, shakiness, perspiration, dizziness, light-headedness, sleepiness, and confusion. If left untreated, hypoglycemia may lead to unconsciousness. *Also known as* insulin reaction.

hypoglycemia unawareness: A state in which a person does not feel or recognize the symptoms of hypoglycemia; common in long-standing diabetes and a risk factor for severe hypoglycemia.

hyponatremia: An abnormally low level of sodium in the blood. This potentially dangerous condition can be caused by burns, vomiting, diarrhea, use of diuretics (especially thiazide diuretics), kidney disease, and congestive heart failure.

hypotension: Low blood pressure or a sudden drop in blood pressure; may occur when a person rises quickly from a seated or reclined position, which can cause dizziness or fainting.

impaired fasting glucose (IFG): A condition in which a fasting plasma glucose test, taken after 8–12 hours of fasting, shows a blood glucose level that is higher than normal but not high enough for a diagnosis of diabetes. People with impaired fasting glucose are at increased risk for developing type 2 diabetes. Also called *prediabetes*.

impaired glucose tolerance (IGT): A condition in which an oral glucose tolerance test shows a blood glucose level higher than normal but not high enough for a diagnosis of diabetes. People with impaired glucose tolerance are at increased risk for developing type 2 diabetes. Also called *prediabetes*.

implantable insulin pump: An insulin pump that is placed inside the body to deliver insulin in response to remote-control commands from the user; currently experimental.

impotence: *See* erectile dysfunction (ED).

incretin: A type of hormone produced by the gut that causes an increase in the amount of insulin released from the beta cells of the islets of the pancreas after eating, even before blood glucose levels become elevated.

incretin mimetic: A class of medications used to treat type 2 diabetes; functions by mimicking (or reproducing) the blood glucose–lowering effects of the naturally occurring incretin hormone. Also called GLP-1 agonists. Generic names: exenatide, liraglutide.

Individualized Education Program (IEP): Under the Individuals with Disabilities in Education Act, a diabetes management plan collaboratively developed by school personnel and the parents of a child with diabetes. Often it is developed based on the child's Diabetes Medical Management Plan. The education plan describes the steps taken to ensure that the student has the same opportunities to participate in all academic and school-sponsored activities while maintaining the student's health; often, this program is more specific than a 504 Plan with regard to the student's academic needs.

Individuals with Disabilities in Education Act (IDEA): A law that guarantees free public education to children with disabilities; children whose diabetes adversely affects their ability to learn generally qualify for protection under this law and often receive an Individualized Education Program (IEP).

inhaled insulin: A rapid-acting insulin that comes in powdered form and is administered through a portable device (called an *inhaler*) that allows a person to breathe in the insulin. Brand name: Afrezza.

injection site: The place on the body where a medication (for example, insulin) is usually injected.

injection site rotation: The process of changing between several different places on the body where an injection is administered; prevents the formation of lipodystrophy.

insoluble fiber: Dietary fiber found in the parts of plants that the body cannot digest (for example, wheat bran and fruit and vegetable skins); aids in the normal functioning of the digestive system.

insulin: A polypeptide hormone that helps the body use glucose for energy; created by the beta cells of the pancreas. All animals (including humans) require insulin to survive. As a medication, it can be taken by injection or pump.

insulin adjustment: The process of changing the amount of insulin a person with diabetes takes based on factors such as meal planning, activity, and blood glucose levels.

insulin analog: A genetically engineered form of insulin that is derived from the human insulin molecule. An analog acts in much the same way as the body's native insulin, but with some beneficial differences for people with diabetes, such as shorter or longer peaks, shorter or longer durations, increased purity, and reduced risk of allergic reactions. Analogs have been developed to serve as basal insulin or bolus insulin.

insulin degludec: An ultra-long-acting basal insulin that is currently available internationally but not yet approved in the United States. As part of a new generation of insulin analogs, it slowly releases insulin into the circulatory system, allowing it to work for a longer period of time. It is an option for patients who need a more flexible insulin regimen. Brand name: Tresiba.

insulin pen: A device for injecting insulin; it resembles a fountain pen and holds cartridges of insulin; a dial is often used to set the insulin dose; most pens are disposable, but some have replaceable cartridges.

insulin pump: An insulin-delivering device about the size of a deck of cards that can be worn on a belt or kept in a pocket. It carries a reservoir of insulin connected to narrow, flexible, plastic tubing that ends with a needle that is inserted just under the skin. Users set the pump to give a basal amount of insulin continuously throughout the day. Pumps also release bolus insulin to cover meals and at times when blood glucose levels are high, based on programming done by the user. Some tubeless or patch pumps are applied directly to the skin and operated by a remote control.

insulin reaction: *See* hypoglycemia.

insulin resistance: A condition characterized by the body's inability to adequately respond to and use insulin, meaning that insulin cannot function properly and higher levels of insulin are needed to achieve the same effects. This can result in high blood glucose levels and high levels of insulin in the blood. If allowed to worsen, prediabetes and type 2 diabetes can develop. Insulin resistance develops in people who have a family history of it, in people who are overweight, and in people who live a sedentary lifestyle.

insulin-to-carbohydrate ratio: A ratio used to determine how many units of bolus insulin a person with diabetes needs to take to cover the effect of carbohydrate on blood glucose levels.

intermediate-acting insulin: A type of insulin that starts to lower blood glucose levels within 1–2 hours after injection and has its strongest effect 6–12 hours after injection. Brand names: ReliOn/Novolin N, Humulin N. *See also* NPH insulin.

intramuscular injection: Inserting liquid medication into a muscle with a syringe. For example, glucagon may be given by intramuscular injection to treat hypoglycemia.

islet cells: Any of the several types of cells located in the pancreas that make hormones to help the body break down and use food for energy. For example, alpha cells make glucagon and beta cells make insulin. *Also known as* islets of Langerhans.

islets of Langerhans: *See* islet cells.

juvenile diabetes: *See* type 1 diabetes.

ketone: A waste product that results from the process of the body breaking down body fat for energy, which is a situation that arises when there is a shortage of insulin. High levels can lead to diabetic ketoacidosis and coma. *Also known as* ketone body.

ketone body: *See* ketone.

ketonuria: A condition occurring when ketones are present in the urine; a warning sign of diabetic ketoacidosis.

ketosis: An elevated level of ketones in the body, which may lead to diabetic ketoacidosis. Signs of ketosis are nausea, vomiting, and stomach pain.

kidney failure: A condition in which the kidneys no longer work properly. There are two types: (1) The chronic condition in which the body retains fluid, causing harmful wastes to build up inside the body. This life-threatening condition is usually treated with dialysis or a kidney transplant. *Also known as* end-stage renal disease. (2) Acute kidney failure (also called *acute renal failure*) that may be caused by sepsis, a bacterial infection, or major blood loss; this may be fatal, yet there is a possibility that damage to the kidneys can be healed and the kidneys fully recover.

Kombiglyze XR: A combination drug that contains saxagliptin (a dipeptidyl peptidase-4 inhibitor) and metformin (a biguanide); used to treat type 2 diabetes.

lactose: A type of sugar found in milk and milk products.

lancet: A small needle used to obtain a drop of blood for blood glucose monitoring.

lancing device: A spring-loaded device used to prick the skin with a small needle to obtain a drop of blood for blood glucose monitoring.

latent autoimmune diabetes in adults (LADA): Autoimmune diabetes that shares many of the characteristics of type 1 diabetes and develops in adults; typically slower in onset than type 1 diabetes in children.

licensed practical nurse (LPN): A nurse who has received 1–2 years of training, received certification and licensing from a state authority, and works under the supervision of registered nurses and physicians. *Also known as* licensed vocational nurse (LVN).

licensed vocational nurse (LVN): *See* licensed practical nurse (LPN).

lifestyle: The way a person or group of people lives; a lifestyle intervention often involves weight loss, diet, and exercise.

linagliptin: An oral hypoglycemic medication used to treat type 2 diabetes and part of the class of medications called dipeptidyl peptidase-4 inhibitors. Brand name: Tradjenta.

lipid: A term for fat in the body, usually broken down by the body and used for energy.

lipid profile: A blood test that measures levels of total cholesterol, triglycerides, LDL cholesterol, and HDL cholesterol. A lipid profile assesses the risk of developing cardiovascular disease.

lipodystrophy: A defect in the breaking down or building up of fat below the surface of the skin, resulting in lumps or small dents in the skin surface; may be caused by repeated injections of insulin in the same spot. Examples include lipohypertrophy and lipoatrophy.

liraglutide: A glucagon-like peptide-1 (GLP-1) agonist that is injected; used to improve blood glucose control in adults with type 2 diabetes. It is not approved for children. Brand name: Victoza.

lispro insulin: A rapid-acting insulin. On average, lispro insulin starts to lower blood glucose levels within 5 minutes after injection and has its strongest effect 30 minutes to 1 hour after injection but keeps working for 3 hours after injection. Brand name: Humalog.

long-acting insulin: A basal insulin that starts to lower blood glucose levels within 4–6 hours after injection and has its strongest effect 10–18 hours after injection. Examples include detemir insulin and glargine insulin.

low-calorie sweetener: A product used to sweeten foods in place of sugar; does not contain many calories per serving and does not raise blood glucose levels. Examples include saccharin, acesulfame-K, aspartame (NutraSweet), and sucralose (Splenda).

low-density lipoprotein (LDL) cholesterol: A fat that travels in the bloodstream; the low-density lipoprotein particle takes cholesterol around the body to where it is needed for cell repair and also deposits it on the inside of artery walls, sometimes leading to atherosclerosis; often called *bad cholesterol* or *unhealthy cholesterol*.

luo han guo fruit extract: A low-calorie natural sweetener that has no nutritional value. It is derived from a plant in Southern China known as monk fruit.

macrovascular disease: Disease of the large blood vessels, such as those found in the heart. Lipids and blood clots build up in the large blood vessels and can cause atherosclerosis, coronary heart disease, stroke, and peripheral vascular disease. *Also known as* cardiovascular disease (CVD).

macular degeneration: An incurable eye disease that affects the *macula* (the central part of the retina) and the central vision. Central vision gives the most direct, focused sight and is needed for the majority of activities, including reading and driving. Macular degeneration is the main cause of vision loss for people aged 55 and older.

managed-care organization: Any type of organization that provides managed care to its members (for example, an exclusive provider organization, health maintenance organization, or preferred provider organization).

mannitol: A sugar alcohol that, when taken in excess, has a laxative effect (causes diarrhea); may be used intravenously to treat increased pressure in the brain.

maturity-onset diabetes of the young (MODY): A rare form of hereditary diabetes that shares the characteristics of type 2 diabetes and generally develops in children or young adults. There are 12 known forms identified; each is caused by a mutation in a different gene and impairs the secretion of insulin. MODY is often misdiagnosed as type 1 diabetes in younger patients and as type 2 diabetes in older patients.

meal plan: A guide to healthy eating for people with diabetes that gives the patient guidance on what to eat, how much to eat, and when to eat; usually developed with the help of a dietitian.

Medicaid: A federal and state healthcare insurance assistance program that is provided to people with very low income or who are disabled or children. The income level at which people can join this program is individually determined by each state.

medical nutrition therapy (MNT): The broad-based approach to adding healthy eating to a person's lifestyle to improve health outcomes; usually includes the development of a meal plan, education in making healthy food choices, and encouraging more physical activity. This is an important part of the process of preventing diabetes, managing existing diabetes, and preventing the rate of development of diabetes complications.

Medicare: A federal healthcare insurance program for people 65 years of age or older and for some people with disabilities who cannot work, as well as people with end-stage renal disease (ESRD). There are two main parts of Medicare: Part A and Part B. Part A helps pay for medical care provided in hospitals, skilled nursing facilities, hospices, and nursing homes. Part B helps pay for health providers' services, ambulance services, diagnostic tests, outpatient hospital services, outpatient physical therapy, speech pathology services, and medical equipment and supplies. In 2005, Part B was updated to include many diabetes-related services, including diabetes screening tests, diabetes self-management education, medical nutrition therapy, and diabetes supplies such as blood glucose monitors, test strips, lancing devices and lancets, control solutions, and sometimes therapeutic shoes. Medicare Part B only covers insulin if it is medically necessary and you use an insulin pump; however, it may be covered under Medicare Part D (prescription drug coverage). Medicare Parts B and D are essential for people with diabetes who qualify for Medicare coverage.

Medigap: An additional healthcare insurance plan that is sold by private insurance companies to pay for some of the costs for which Medicare does not provide coverage (thus, it pays for the "gaps" in Medicare coverage). The policies must follow federal and state laws and be identified as Medicare Supplement Insurance. Plans vary from one insurance company to another, so consumers have to carefully evaluate the benefits of individual Medigap plans.

meglitinide: A class of oral medicine for type 2 diabetes; lowers blood glucose levels by helping the pancreas make more insulin after meals. Generic name: repaglinide.

metabolic syndrome: A collection of various risk factors that tend to group together in individuals (including obesity, high blood glucose, hypertension, and dyslipidemia) and can lead to heart disease. This is not necessarily a disease that is diagnosed; instead, it's a tool for estimating the risk of the development of heart disease.

metabolism: The umbrella term for the way cells chemically change food so it can be used to store or burn energy and make the proteins, fats, and sugars needed by the body.

metformin: An oral medicine belonging to the biguanide class of medications used to treat type 2 diabetes. Brand names: Glucophage, Glucophage XR.

microvascular disease: Disease of the smallest blood vessels, such as those found in the eyes, nerves, and kidneys. The walls of the vessels become abnormally thick but weak, and then they may bleed, leak protein, and slow the flow of blood to the cells.

miglitol: An oral medicine used to treat type 2 diabetes and belonging to the class of medicines called *alpha-glucosidase inhibitors.* Brand name: Glyset.

mixed dose: A combination of two types of insulin in one injection. Typically, a rapid- or short-acting insulin is combined with a longer-acting insulin (such as NPH insulin) to provide both mealtime and basal management of blood glucose levels.

monounsaturated fat: A type of "healthy" dietary fat that is found in some foods from plants, particularly olive and canola oils, and including avocados, nuts, and peanut butter; usually in liquid form when at room temperature.

morbid obesity: Severe obesity in which a person has a BMI over 40 kg/m^2; usually equivalent to being 100 pounds over ideal body weight.

morbidity: The state of being ill or diseased; any departure from overall health.

mortality: A measure of the rate of death in total or from a particular disease within a given population.

nateglinide: An oral medicine used to treat type 2 diabetes; belongs to the class of medicines called d-phenylalanine derivatives. Brand name: Starlix.

neotame: A low-calorie artificial sweetener with few calories and no nutritional value; a modified form of aspartame. Approved in the United States in 2002. It is mainly used in the production of food. Brand name: Newtame.

nephrologist: A doctor who treats people who have kidney problems.

nephropathy: Disease of the kidneys. Hyperglycemia and hypertension can damage the glomerulus of the kidney. When the kidneys are damaged, protein leaks into the urine. If damage progresses, the kidneys can no longer remove waste and extra fluids from the bloodstream.

neurologist: A doctor who specializes in problems of the nervous system, such as neuropathy or stroke.

neuropathy: Disease of the nervous system; a complication of diabetes. The three major forms in people with diabetes are peripheral neuropathy, autonomic neuropathy, and mononeuropathy. The most common form is peripheral neuropathy, which primarily affects the legs and feet.

N insulin: *See* NPH insulin.

non–insulin-dependent diabetes mellitus (NIDDM): *See* type 2 diabetes.

non-proliferative retinopathy: *See* background diabetic retinopathy.

nontropical sprue: *See* celiac disease.

NPH insulin: An intermediate-acting insulin; NPH stands for neutral protamine Hagedorn. Protamine is a protein that, when added to regular insulin, slows down its onset and prolongs its duration. NPH insulin starts to lower blood glucose within 1–2 hours after injection and has its strongest effect 6–10 hours after injection but keeps working for about 10 hours after injection. *Also known as* N insulin. *See also* intermediate-acting insulin.

nurse practitioner (NP): A registered nurse who has taken advanced training and received a master's degree in nursing; can perform many of the duties of a physician without direct supervision; may take on additional duties in diagnosis and treatment of patients.

Nutrition Facts label: A standardized label on any food or beverage providing nutritional information that is required on any food distributed in the United States. The Nutrition Facts label is regulated by the U.S. Food and Drug Administration. This label must contain the following information: serving size, servings per container, calories, calories from fat, total fat, saturated fat, trans fat, cholesterol, sodium, total carbohydrate, dietary fiber, sugars, and protein. The label may also include calcium, iron, vitamin A, and vitamin C. For many elements, it assumes that 2,000 calories are being consumed in a day, and the percentages given reflect how much the food item delivers.

nutritionist: A person with training in nutrition; may or may not have specialized training and qualifications.

nutrition therapy: *See* medical nutrition therapy.

Obamacare: *See* Affordable Care Act.

obese: An abnormally high, unhealthy body weight; defined as a body mass index of 30 kg/m² or higher.

omega-3 fatty acid: A polyunsaturated fat that is mainly found in oily, fatty fish, such as wild salmon, herring, tuna, and anchovies; also found in flaxseed oil; has an anti-inflammatory effect and may be beneficial to heart health. Also written as ω-3 *fatty acid.*

ophthalmologist: A medical doctor who diagnoses and treats all eye diseases and eye disorders; can also prescribe glasses and contact lenses.

optometrist: A primary eye care provider who prescribes glasses and contact lenses; can diagnose and treat certain eye conditions and diseases.

oral glucose tolerance test (OGTT): A test to diagnose diabetes, gestational diabetes, or impaired glucose tolerance; administered after an overnight fast. A blood sample is taken and then the patient drinks a high-glucose beverage. Blood samples are then taken at intervals for 2–3 hours.

oral hypoglycemic agent: Medicine taken by mouth to treat high blood glucose; generally prescribed to treat type 2 diabetes. Classes of this medication include alpha-glucosidase inhibitors, biguanides, d-phenylalanine derivatives, meglitinides, sulfonyl-ureas, thiazolidinediones, DPP-4 inhibitors, SGLT2 inhibitors, and others.

overweight: An above-normal body weight, but not obese; defined as a body mass index of 25–29.9 kg/m^2.

pancreas: A comma-shaped gland located just behind the stomach that produces enzymes for digesting food and hormones that regulate the use of fuels in the body, including insulin and glucagon.

pediatric endocrinologist: A doctor who treats children who have endocrine gland problems such as diabetes.

pedorthist: A healthcare professional who specializes in fitting shoes for people with disabilities or deformities and can make custom shoes or orthotics (for example, special inserts for shoes).

periodontist: A dentist who specializes in treating people who have gum diseases.

peripheral arterial disease (PAD): A disease that occurs when blood vessels in the legs are narrowed or blocked by fatty deposits, reducing blood flow to the feet and legs. This condition can cause *claudication* (pain with walking) and puts people at increased risk of foot problems such as gangrene. One out of every three people with diabetes aged 50 years or older is estimated to have this condition. *Also known as* peripheral vascular disease (PVD).

peripheral neuropathy: Nerve damage that affects the feet, legs, or hands; causes pain, numbness, or a tingling feeling. *Also known as* distal symmetric polyneuropathy.

peripheral vascular disease (PVD): *See* peripheral arterial disease (PAD).

pharmacist: A healthcare professional who prepares and distributes medicine to people. Pharmacists also give information on medicines.

physical activity: Any form of exercise or movement, including walking, running, sports, and regular day-to-day activities, such as yard work, walking the dog, cleaning, and running errands. Adults should try to get at least 30 minutes of moderate physical activity (any activity that requires about as much energy as brisk walking) at least 5 days a week.

physician assistant: A healthcare professional who is trained and licensed to practice medicine under the guidance of a supervising physician.

pioglitazone: An oral medicine used to treat type 2 diabetes; belongs to the class of medicines called thiazolidinediones. Brand name: Actos.

podiatrist: A healthcare professional who treats people who have foot problems; also helps people keep their feet healthy by providing regular foot examinations and treatment.

polydipsia: Excessive thirst; may be a sign of uncontrolled diabetes.

polyol: *See* sugar alcohol.

polyphagia: Excessive hunger; may be a sign of uncontrolled diabetes.

polyunsaturated fat: A type of "healthy" dietary fat that is found in large amounts in some foods from plants, particularly vegetable oils, such as those from safflower, sunflower, cottonseed, soybean, and corn; can also be found in margarine; usually in liquid form when at room temperature.

polyuria: Excessive urination; may be a sign of uncontrolled diabetes.

portion control: The process of eating sensible serving sizes; essential for achieving weight loss and maintaining a healthy body weight; a key tactic in meal planning.

postprandial: After a meal. A postprandial blood glucose level is one taken 1–2 hours after eating.

pramlintide: An injectable medication for the treatment of diabetes; it is a synthetic form of the hormone amylin. Pramlintide injections taken with meals have been shown to modestly improve A1C levels without causing increased hypoglycemia or weight gain and even promote slight weight loss. The primary side effect is nausea, which tends to improve over time and as an individual patient determines his or her optimal dose. Brand name: Symlin.

prediabetes: A condition in which blood glucose levels are higher than normal but are not high enough for a diagnosis of diabetes. People with prediabetes are at increased risk for developing type 2 diabetes and for heart disease and stroke. Subtypes are called *impaired glucose tolerance* and *impaired fasting glucose.*

preferred provider organization (PPO): A managed-care plan that arranges coverage for specific services through a network of participating providers that is contracted by the insurance company. Under this type of plan, most healthcare costs are covered when a network physician is visited.

premixed insulin: A commercially produced combination of two different types of insulin. Examples include 50/50 insulin, 75/25 insulin, and 70/30 insulin.

preprandial: Before a meal.

proliferative retinopathy: A condition in which fragile new blood vessels grow along the retina, which can cause blood to leak into the clear fluid inside the eye and can also cause the retina to detach; sometimes leads to loss of vision (blindness).

protein: (1) One of the main nutrients in food. Foods that provide protein include meat, poultry, fish, dairy products, eggs, and dried beans. (2) Chains of amino acids produced by the body to build cell structure, make hormones such as insulin, and for other various functions.

proteinuria: The presence of protein in the urine, indicating that the kidneys are not working properly.

psychiatrist: A medical doctor who specializes in the evaluation, diagnosis, and treatment of mental disorders; can prescribe medications.

psychologist: A healthcare professional who treats people through counseling in an attempt to help overcome emotional or psychological reactions to injury, disease, or other experiences; cannot prescribe medications.

random plasma glucose test: A test in which blood is drawn at any point in the day, regardless of whether the subject is fasting, to determine blood glucose levels; if blood glucose levels are abnormal, a fasting plasma glucose test or A1C test may be used to diagnose diabetes. *Also known as* casual plasma glucose test.

rapid-acting insulin: A type of insulin that starts to lower blood glucose levels within 5–10 minutes after injection and has its strongest effect about 90 minutes to 2 hours after injection. Examples include aspart insulin, lispro insulin, and glulisine insulin.

rebound hyperglycemia: A swing to high blood glucose levels after hypoglycemia. *Also known as* Somogyi effect.

Recognized Diabetes Education Program: Diabetes self-management education program that meets the American Diabetes Association's National Standards for Diabetes Self-Management Education.

Recommended Dietary Allowance (RDA): One of the four reference values of the Dietary Reference Intake; the average daily intake level that is sufficient to meet the nutrient requirements of nearly all healthy individuals of a particular age and gender.

registered dietitian nutritionist (RDN): An expert on the science of food and nutrition who promotes healthy living. RDNs work with hospitals, schools, public health clinics, nursing homes, fitness centers, the food industry, research institutions, healthcare private practices, and universities. RDNs have completed a bachelor's degree from a university or college approved by the Accreditation Council for Education in Nutrition and Dietetics (ACEND) of the Academy of Nutrition and Dietetics, completed an approved practice program, and passed the national exam administered by the Commission on Dietetic Registration. These professionals have formerly been called registered dietitians (RDs).

registered nurse (RN): A nurse who has taken 2 or more years of education and training in providing nursing care and passed a board examination.

regular insulin: A short-acting insulin that is molecularly identical to insulin produced by the body. On average, regular insulin starts to lower blood glucose levels within 30 minutes after injection under the skin and has its strongest effect 2–5 hours after injection but keeps working for 5–8 hours after injection. Sometimes it's given intravenously in hospital settings. *Also known as* R insulin *and* short-acting insulin.

repaglinide: An oral medicine used to treat type 2 diabetes and belonging to the class of medicines called meglitinides. Brand name: Prandin.

retinopathy: Damage to small blood vessels in the eye that can lead to vision problems; different forms include background retinopathy and proliferative retinopathy.

R insulin: *See* regular insulin.

risk factor: Anything that raises the chances of a person developing a disease.

rosiglitazone: An oral medicine used to treat type 2 diabetes and belonging to the class of medicines called thiazolidinediones. Brand name: Avandia.

Rule of 15: *See* 15-gram/15-minute rule.

saccharin: An artificial sweetener with no calories and no nutritional value. Brand names: Sweet'N Low, Sugar Twin, Necta Sweet.

saturated fat: A fat found mainly in animal-based foods, such as meat and dairy products, but also in some oils, such as palm oil and coconut oil; can raise LDL cholesterol levels; is often a solid fat when at room temperature.

saxagliptin: An oral hypoglycemic agent used to treat type 2 diabetes and belonging to the class of medications called dipeptidyl peptidase-4 inhibitors. Brand name: Onglyza.

secondary diabetes: A type of diabetes that develops because of the effects of another disease or because of reactions to certain drugs or chemicals.

sedentary lifestyle: A way of life characterized by a lack of physical activity.

self-monitoring of blood glucose (SMBG): The process by which a person with diabetes checks, records, and evaluates his or her own blood glucose levels; an essential component of pattern management and the key to diabetes self-care.

serving size: (1) The size of a portion of food that is eaten in one sitting; in many cases, people eat meals in which the serving size is too large, contributing to being overweight or obese. (2) A listing on a Nutrition Facts label that identifies how much of a certain food constitutes one serving.

short-acting insulin: A type of insulin that starts to lower blood glucose levels within 30 minutes after injection and has its strongest effect 2–5 hours after injection. *Also known as* regular insulin.

sitagliptin: An oral hypoglycemic agent used to treat type 2 diabetes and belonging to the class of medications called dipeptidyl peptidase-4 inhibitors. Brand name: Januvia.

sodium: A mineral and dietary nutrient that helps maintain the balance of water in the cells and keeps nerves functioning. Most excess dietary sodium comes in the form of table salt or salt added to processed foods; in excess, it can contribute to high blood pressure.

sodium-glucose cotransporter 2 inhibitor (SGLT2): A medication used to treat type 2 diabetes. SGLT2 is a protein involved in the absorption of glucose in the kidneys. An SGLT2 inhibitor stops SGLT2 from working and therefore increases the amount of glucose released through the urine. This lowers the blood glucose levels. Brand names: Invokana, Farxiga, Jardiance.

soluble fiber: Dietary fiber found in foods such as oats, barley, fruits, and vegetables; can help improve serum lipid levels.

Somogyi effect: *See* rebound hyperglycemia.

sorbitol: (1) A sugar alcohol (sweetener) with 2.6 calories per gram. (2) A substance produced by the body when blood glucose levels are high that can cause damage to the eyes and nerves.

split mixed dose: Two types of insulin mixed in the same syringe and given two or more times over the course of the day.

starch: One of the three main types of carbohydrate; dietary sources include beans, lentils, grains, breads, and starchy vegetables (such as peas, potatoes, and corn). *Also known as* complex carbohydrate.

steviol glycoside: A low-calorie, artificial sweetener with no nutritional value; derived from the stevia plant in South America. Brand name: Truvia.

strength training: Activities specifically designed to build muscle and increase strength.

stretching: *See* flexibility exercise.

subcutaneous (SC): Under the skin. Fluid that is subcutaneous has glucose levels similar to blood and is what a continuous glucose monitor (CGM) measures. Insulin and some other medications are injected subcutaneously.

sucralose: An artificial, low-calorie sweetener with no nutritional value. Brand name: Splenda.

sucrose: A simple sugar that the body breaks down into glucose and fructose; also known as *table sugar* or *white sugar,* it is found naturally in sugar cane and in beets.

sugar alcohol: A sweetener that produces a smaller rise in blood glucose than other carbohydrates; contains about 2 calories per gram; includes erythritol, isomalt, lactitol, maltitol, mannitol, sorbitol, and xylitol. *Also known as* polyol.

sugar substitute: A substance used to sweeten foods; used in place of sugar. Some sugar substitutes have calories and will affect blood glucose levels, such as fructose and sugar alcohols (for example, sorbitol and mannitol). Others have very few calories and will not affect blood glucose levels, such as the low-calorie sweeteners, saccharin, acesulfame-K, aspartame (NutraSweet), sucralose (Splenda), and stevia (Truvia).

sulfonylurea: A class of oral medication for type 2 diabetes that lowers blood glucose levels by stimulating the beta cells to make more insulin. The most common side effect of this class of drug is hypoglycemia. Generic names: glimepiride, glipizide, glyburide.

team management: A diabetes treatment approach in which medical care is provided by a healthcare team, usually consisting of a doctor, a dietitian, a nurse, a diabetes educator, and others. The team acts as advisers to the person with diabetes.

telehealth: *See* telemedicine.

telemedicine: The use of telecommunications technologies (such as telephones, videoconferencing, and the Internet) to deliver medical care from a distance, particularly medical diagnoses, patient care, and consultations; especially useful in rural areas, where access to certain types of advanced care may not be readily available or nearby. *Also known as* telehealth.

thiazide diuretic: A class of antihypertensive drug. Examples include hydrochlorothiazide (HCTZ).

thiazolidinedione: A class of oral medicine for type 2 diabetes that helps insulin take glucose from the blood into the cells for energy by making cells more sensitive to insulin. Generic names: pioglitazone, rosiglitazone.

Tolerable Upper Intake Level (UL): One of the four reference values of the Dietary Reference Intake; the highest level of daily intake of a nutrient that will likely not increase the risk of developing an adverse health effect. If intake increases beyond the Tolerable Upper Intake Level, then the risk of adverse effects increases.

trans fat: *See* trans fatty acid.

trans fatty acid: A fat that is produced when liquid fat (oil) is turned into solid fat through a chemical process called *hydrogenation;* found in foods such as margarine, shortening, and baked foods (for example, cookies, crackers, muffins, and cereals). Eating a large amount of trans fatty acids can raise LDL cholesterol, thus increasing the risk of heart disease. The U.S. Food and Drug Administration (FDA) requires that trans fatty acids be listed on the Nutrition Facts label of every food. Some states and cities in the United States have also banned restaurants from serving foods that contain trans fatty acids. *Also known as* trans fat.

triglyceride: The storage form of fat in the body; circulates in the blood and is measured as part of a lipid profile or panel. Blood levels may be high in type 2 diabetes.

type 1 diabetes (T1DM, T1D): A less common form of diabetes mellitus than type 2. Once called juvenile diabetes, it is characterized by high blood glucose levels caused by a total lack of insulin. It occurs when the body's immune system attacks the insulin-producing beta cells in the pancreas and destroys them; the pancreas then produces little or no insulin. Type 1 diabetes develops most often in young people but can appear in adults. It is primarily treated with insulin therapy, meal planning, exercise, and self-monitoring of blood glucose.

type 2 diabetes (T2DM, T2D): The most common form of diabetes mellitus; characterized by high blood glucose levels caused by a relative lack of insulin or the body's inability to properly use insulin (insulin resistance) or both. Type 2 diabetes develops most often in middle-aged and older adults but can appear in young people; most people who develop this disease are overweight or obese. It is primarily treated with meal planning, exercise, oral hypoglycemic agents, self-monitoring of blood glucose, and insulin therapy.

unit of insulin: The basic measure of the biological effects of a standardized amount of insulin; equal to 45.5 micrograms of pure, crystallized insulin; sometimes presented as 1 international unit, 1 IU, or 1 UI. Insulin is dosed in units. Most insulin preparations are U-100, meaning there are 100 units of insulin per milliliter of solution.

urine testing: A test of a urine sample used to diagnose diseases of the urinary system and other body systems; may also check for signs of bleeding; for people with diabetes, used to check for the presence of ketones, albumin, or (less frequently) glucose.

urologist: A doctor who treats people who have urinary tract problems; also cares for men who have problems with their genital organs, such as erectile dysfunction.

vaccination: A process of immunization that is intended to confer resistance to a specific disease; conducted by administering a weakened or inactive form of a disease to provoke an immune response that will provide defense against a more serious form of the disease. This procedure works because the human immune system can develop the ability to quickly respond to a disease after it has been exposed to it before.

very-low-density lipoprotein (VLDL) cholesterol: A cholesterol found in a particle that transports triglycerides in the blood; some of this is converted to LDL cholesterol; high levels may be related to cardiovascular disease.

vildagliptin: An oral hypoglycemic agent used to treat type 2 diabetes and belonging to the dipeptidyl peptidase-4 inhibitor class of medications. Brand name: Galvus.

waist circumference: The measurement of the size of the waist; used to estimate the risks of a person developing obesity-related health problems. Women with a waist measurement of more than 35 inches or men with a waist measurement of more than 40 inches have a higher risk of developing diabetes, hypertension, and heart disease; the waist measurements that indicate risk may be lower in Asians.

whole grain: A food in which the whole kernels of a grain (for example, barley, corn, oats, wheat, rye) are used; believed to provide greater health benefits because it contains dietary fiber, antioxidants, minerals, and vitamins. Common whole-grain products include oatmeal, popcorn, brown rice, whole-wheat flour, and whole-wheat bread.

xylitol: A carbohydrate-based sugar alcohol that is found in plants and used as a sugar substitute; provides calories; added to some mints and chewing gum.

Index

A

A1C test, 14, 15, 21, 38, 44, 56, 266

AADE (American Association of Diabetes Educators), 50, 52

AAP (American Academy of Pediatrics), 215, 216

Academy of Nutrition and Dietetics, 31, 132, 166

acarbose (Precose), 58, 61

ACCORD study, 263

ACE inhibitors, 75, 260

acesulfame potassium (Sunett, Sweet One), 142, 265

activity monitors, 189–190

acute, defined, 265

added sugars, 149, 150, 223

Adequate Intake (AI), 265

adipose tissue, 265

adult-onset diabetes, former name for type 2 diabetes, 213

advantame, 142, 265

aerobic exercise, 178, 183, 186, 265

Affordable Care Act (ACA) (Obamacare), 230, 265

agave nectar, 143

age, as risk factor, 15

airport security, preparing for, 247–248

albiglutide (Tanzeum), 266

albumin, 106, 266

albumin excretion rate (AER), 266

albuminuria, 266

alcohol, 153, 197, 219

alogliptin (Nesina), 58, 60, 266

alogliptin and pioglitazone (Oseni), 63

alpha cells, 8

alpha-glucosidase inhibitors, 58, 61, 266

American Academy of Pediatrics (AAP), 215, 216

American Association of Diabetes Educators (AADE), 50, 52

American College of Sports Medicine, 33

American Diabetes Association

A1C recommendation, 260

A1C recommendation during pregnancy, 115

A1C recommendation for children and teens, 215

"Be Healthy Today; Be Healthy For Life," 217

booklet of food lists, 166

on consumption of carbohydrates, 137

on consumption of fats, 144

on consumption of omega-3 fats, 145

on consumption of proteins, 143

on counting calories, 136

Diabetes Forecast, 72, 88, 203, 207, 209

events hosted by, 202

on fish oil supplements, 151

guidelines about metabolic surgery, 77

help in locating diabetes education programs, 52–53

for information on understanding rights, 243

on meal plans, 164, 166, 169

message boards on, 21

on nonnutritive sweeteners, 142

on omega-3 supplements, 151

purpose of, 2

for recipes and cookbooks, 171

American Diabetes Association (continued)

recognition by of first digital program (One Drop-Experts), 51

recommendation for aerobic exercise, 183, 184

recommendation for breastfeeding, 118

recommendation for dilated eye exams, 262, 263

recommendation for exercise, 186, 187

recommendation for flexibility and balance exercises, 185

recommendation for resistance exercise, 184

recommendation for sitting less and moving more, 180

recommendation for sodium consumption, 151

recommendation for taking statins, 75

recommendation for testing of children, 215

recommended blood glucose level, 260

recommended blood glucose targets, 84

recommended blood pressure level, 260

recommended fasting blood glucose level, 260

recommended weight gain during pregnancy, 115

on rights as person with diabetes, 241

on sugar-sweetened drinks, 141

on type 2 diabetes as not a choice, 221

vaccination recommendations, 42

website. See diabetes.org (website)

as working with Transportation Security Administration (TSA), 247

American Heart Association, 141, 223

American Society of Exercise Physiologists, 33

American Stroke Association, 99

Americans with Disabilities Act, 243, 246, 266

Americans with Disabilities Act Amendments Acts of 2008, 243

amputation, 19, 40, 103, 104, 226

amylin, 63, 64, 266

amylin analogs, 63, 64

analog, defined, 266

analog insulin, 66, 67–69

anger, 195

angiopathy, 266

angiotensin, 266

angiotensin II receptor blockers (ARBs), 75, 260, 266

ankle-brachial index test, 44, 105

antidepressants, 106, 108, 124, 200, 201

anti-discrimination laws, 243, 245–246

antihypertensive drug, 266

antioxidants, 157, 158, 266

anti-VEGF injections, 263

anxiety disorders, 200–201

Apple, apps to track movements, 190

apps

for exercise, 189–190

for fun ways to work out, 255–256

to help track blood glucose data, 89

for telling you calories and nutrition information for foods, 136

ARBs (angiotensin II receptor blockers), 75, 260, 266

arteries, hardening of, 98–99

artificial pancreas, 74

artificial sweeteners, 142–143

aspart insulin (Novolog), 68, 266

aspartame (Equal, Nutrasweet), 142, 266

aspirin, use of, 75–76

atherosclerosis, 98, 127

atorvastatin (Lipitor), 75

audio features, on blood glucose meter, 86

autonomic body systems, 91

autonomic neuropathy, 105, 106, 267

B

C

calcium, 149, 150

calcium channel blocker (CCB), 75, 268

calluses, protecting feet from, 103

calories, 135–136, 148, 178

canagliflozin (Invokana), 58, 61

Candida albicans, 120

cannula, 73

capillaries, 261

carbohydrates
  basics of, 137–138
  counting of, 167–169, 268
  defined, 268
  as listed on food labels, 149
  listing of, 167–168
  as one of three main groups of nutrients, 137
  portion matters with, 168
  reading food labels for, 168–169
  types of, 138–141

cardiometabolic risk factors, 268

cardiometabolic syndrome, 99

cardiovascular disease (CVD), 11, 61, 64, 74, 75, 76, 98, 143, 145, 149, 158, 164, 166, 187, 197, 218, 232, 268

caregivers, tips for, 209–211

casual plasma glucose test, 268

cataracts, 102, 260, 261, 262, 263

CCB (calcium channel blocker), 75, 268

celiac disease/celiac sprue, 268

Centers for Disease Control and Prevention, 42, 53, 213, 226, 244

Centers for Medicare and Medicaid Services, 231

certified diabetes educator (CDE), 21, 29–30, 50, 133, 268

certified dietitian nutritionist (CDN), 132

CGM (continuous glucose monitor), 73, 74, 85, 269

CHD (coronary heart disease), 262, 269

Cheat Sheet, 3

checkups
  for children/teens with type 2 diabetes, 218
  importance of communication at, 45
  making time for yearly eye exam, 43
  overview of, 44
  what to bring with you to, 44–45
  what to expect in, 37–43

children, raising of with type 2 diabetes, 213–220, 245–246

Children's Health Insurance Program (CHIP), 233

chocolate, myth of people with diabetes not able to eat, 222–223

cholesterol. *See also* bad cholesterol; good cholesterol; high-density lipoprotein (HDL) cholesterol; low-density lipoprotein (LDL) cholesterol
  defined, 41, 144
  as listed on food labels, 149
  lowering of to keep eyes healthy, 260
  medication to treat, 75
  targets for, 40–41
  testing of, 44
  types of, 41

Choose Your Foods: Food Lists for Diabetes (American Diabetes Association and Academy of Nutrition and Dietetics), 166

choosemyplate.gov (website), 164

chromium, 151

chronic, 268

Cialis, 125

clinical psychologist, role of, 35

COBRA (Consolidated Omnibus Budget Reconciliation Act), 269

coffee, 152

cognitive behavioral therapy, 201

co-insurance, 268

Colberg, Sheri R. (author)
  Diabetes & Keeping Fit For Dummies, 178

dumping syndrome, 77

dyslipidemia, 271

E

eAG (estimated average glucose), 38, 271

EAR (Estimate Average Requirement), 271

Eat Out, Eat Well (Warshaw), 174

eating out with confidence, 133, 174–175. *See also* restaurants

eatright.org (website), 31

ED (erectile dysfunction), 124–126, 271

education and empowerment, gaining of, 203

eGFR (estimated glomerular filtration rate), 107, 272

eGFR (serum creatinine), 41, 44

800-DIABETES (800-342-2383), 243

800-QUIT-NOW, 261

eldercare.gov (website), 239

emergencies, talking about with your family, 207

emergency room (ER) visits, 237–238

emotions

being kind to yourself, 202–204

being mindful of, 108–109

connecting with others in online support groups, 202

gaining education and empowerment, 203

getting in touch with how you feel, 194

joining local support group, 201–202

looking at depression and anxiety disorders, 199–201

managing of, 193–204

managing stress, 196–198

minding of, 35

reaching out to others, 201–202

recognizing diabetes distress and burnout, 198–199

taking time for yourself, 203

trying mindfulness and meditation, 203–204

empagliflozin (Jardiance), 58, 61

empagliflozin and linagliptin (Glyxambi), 63

employer-based health insurance, 231

endocrinologist, 26, 271

endorphins, 18, 179, 188

epidemiology, 271

erectile dysfunction (ED), 124–126, 271

Estimate Average Requirement (EAR), 271

estimated average glucose (eAG), 38, 271

estimated glomerular filtration rate (eGFR), 107, 272

estrogen, 112

ethnicity, as risk factor, 15, 214, 215

exclusive provider organization (EPO), 272

exenatide (Byetta), 63, 64, 272

exercise

benefits of, 11, 18, 22, 75, 178–179

boosting mood with, 188

checking blood glucose during, 181

with children/teens with type 2 diabetes, 217

completing well-rounded workout, 185–187

dancing, 258

defined, 184

envisioning health benefits of, 187–188

first steps to, 179–182

fitness goals, 181–182, 186, 187, 189

flexibility exercise, 273

focusing on with children/teens to manage condition, 215–216

fun ways to work out for people who hate to exercise, 253–258

getting a buddy for, 254

getting detailed feedback from fitness trackers and apps, 189–190

getting help from professional, 188

getting muscles moving, 180–181

getting support from friends and family, 189

as improving insulin sensitivity, 10

incorporating fun into, 180

exercise *(continued)*

  a.k.a. physical activity, 177

  as mood booster, 18

  motivators to keep you going, 187–190

  playing like a kid, 254–255

  during pregnancy, 115

  setting goals for, 39, 257–258

  strength training, 183

  talking to healthcare provider about, 181

  thinking positive thoughts, 256

  turning up the volume, 256

  types of, 182–185

  volunteering to help someone else, 257

  walking, 180, 255

  walking to raise money, 257

exercise physiologist, 33, 188, 272

extended release exenatide (Bydureon), 63, 64

eye diseases, 261–262

EyeCare America, 236

eyes. *See also* dilated eye exam

  checking of during pregnancy, 115

  consideration of during pregnancy, 263

  getting the treatment you need, 262

  importance of getting regular dilated eye exams, 262–263

  making time for yearly eye exam, 43

  parts of, 102

  taking care of, 31–32, 101–102

  things to do for yours, 259–264

F

family

  changes in with children/teens with type 2 diabetes, 216–217

  educating yours about your diagnosis, 206–207

  exercising with, 209

  making healthy food choices together, 208

  opening lines of communication with, 207–208

  talking to about emergencies, 207

  turning to for support, 206–209

family history, as risk factor, 15, 214, 215, 264

Family Medical Leave Act (FMLA), 243, 246

family therapist, role of, 36

FAST acronym (stroke symptoms), 99

fast-acting insulin, 68

fasting plasma glucose (FPG) test, 14, 15, 272

fats, 137, 144–146, 149, 272. *See also* monounsaturated fats; omega-3 fats/omega-3 fatty acid; polyunsaturated fats; saturated fats; trans fats; unsaturated fats

FDA (Food and Drug Administration), 57, 62, 64, 85–86, 142, 147, 149, 159

feedback, from fitness trackers and apps, 189

fee-for-service healthcare, 272

feet, 34–35, 42, 103–105, 248

15-gram/15-minute rule, 93–94, 272

50/50 insulin, 272

50% lispro protamine (NPL)/50% lispro (Humalog Mix 50/50), 68

fitness instructors, 33

fitness professionals, 188

fitness trackers, 189–190

504 Plan, 246, 272

flexibility exercise, 183, 185, 273

flu, myth of people with diabetes as more likely to get, 224–225

flu shot/flu vaccine, 42, 224

FMLA (Family Medical Leave Act), 243, 246

focal neuropathy, 273

Food and Drug Administration (FDA), 57, 62, 64, 85–86, 142, 147, 149, 159

Food Composition Databases (USDA), 136

food labels, 146, 147–150, 168–169

food list, 165

making healthy food choices together with family, 208

meal plans that work for you, 162–163

Mediterranean-style eating plan (Mediterranean diet), 164–165

planning ones, 155–175

planning smart, 170–171

recipes, 171, 208, 209

shopping smart, 171–172

tempting taste buds with nutritious nibbles, 172–174

turning to dietitian for help, 163–164

weighing and measuring food, 160–161

while traveling, 248

working with a dietitian, 30–31

heart

maintaining healthy heart, 98–99

men as needing to pay attention to heart health, 127

women as needing to pay particular attention to, 122

heart attacks, 11, 40, 64, 97, 98, 99, 122, 127, 162

heart disease, 11, 16, 19, 41, 65, 74, 75, 95, 98, 99, 108, 111, 122, 127, 132, 144, 145, 164, 178, 181, 224, 226, 256, 257, 275

heart rate, measurement of, 186–187, 190

height, measurement of at checkups, 39

hemoglobin, 14, 275

hemorrhagic stroke, 99

hepatitis B vaccine, 42

HHS (hyperosmolar hyperglycemic syndrome), 97, 275

high blood glucose, 10–11, 18, 20, 56, 91, 95–97, 104. *See also* hyperglycemia

high blood pressure, 11, 16, 40, 41

high-contrast screen, on blood glucose meter, 86

high-density lipoprotein (HDL) cholesterol, 41, 75, 275. *See also* good cholesterol

high-fructose corn syrup, 142

HIPPA (Health Insurance Portability and Accountability Act), 275

HMO (health maintenance organization), 275

holidays, celebrating of, 176

home healthcare, 239

honeymoon phase, 275

hormone replacement therapy (HRT), 119

hospital stays, 237, 238–239

hot flashes, 120

human insulin, 67

hybrid closed-loop system, 74

hyperglycemia, 90, 95, 96, 260, 275

hyperinsulinemia, 275

hyperlipidemia, 275

hypernatremia, 275

hyperosmolar hyperglycemic syndrome (HHS), 97, 275

hypertension, 99, 276

hypoglycemia, 61, 90, 92, 117, 181, 207, 219, 244, 276

hypoglycemia unawareness, 93, 276

hyponatremia, 276

I

icons, explained, 3

ID bracelet, 238

impaired fasting glucose (IFG), 276

impaired glucose tolerance (IGT), 276

implantable insulin pump, 276

incretin mimetics, 64, 276

incretins, 60, 276

individual health insurance, 234

Individualized Education Program (IEP), 218, 276

Individuals with Disabilities Education Act (IDEA), 246, 277

inhaled insulin (Afrezza), 68, 69, 277

injected medications (besides insulin), 63–64

nephrologist, 36, 281

nephropathy, 282

nerves, 105–106

neurologist, 282

neuropathy, 105, 106, 124, 282

newborns, testing of, 117

night sweats, 120

nonstarchy vegetables, 138–139

NPH (intermediate-acting insulin), 67, 68, 278

NPH insulin

  Humulin N, 68

  a.k.a. N insulin, 282

  Novolin N, 68

nurse practitioner (NP), 26, 282

nursing home, 239

nutrients

  to avoid, 150

  carbohydrates, 137–143

  to embrace, 150

  fats, 144–146

  as listed on food labels, 148–149

  proteins, 143–144

nutrition, 131–153, 215–216

Nutrition Facts label, 282

nutritionist, 282

nutritious nibbles, 172–174

O

obese, defined, 282

obesity, 214, 217

omega-3 fats/omega-3 fatty acid, 145, 283

One Drop-Experts (app), 51

online support groups, 202, 217

ophthalmologist, 31–32, 43, 44, 283

optometrist, 31–32, 43, 44, 283

oral care, importance of, 33

oral glucose tolerance test (OGTT), 13, 14, 15, 283

oral hygiene hints, 101

oral hypoglycemic agent, 283

oral medications, pills for type 2 diabetes, 57–63

orlistat (Alli, Xenical), 76

over-the-counter medications, 32, 57

overweight, defined, 283

P

PAD (peripheral arterial disease/peripheral artery disease), 41, 44, 104–105, 283

paleo diet, 166

pancreas, 8, 9, 74, 283

Partnership for Prescription Assistance, 236

PAs (physician assistants), 26, 284

Patient Access Network Foundation, 236

PCOS (polycystic ovary syndrome), 114

PCV13 vaccine, 42

pediatric endocrinologist, 283

pedorhist, 283

peeing, as symptom of high blood glucose, 10

pens, for injecting insulin, 69, 70–71, 277

percent daily value, as listed on food labels, 149

perimenopause, 118

periodontist, 283

peripheral (side) vision, 262

peripheral arterial disease/peripheral artery disease (PAD), 41, 44, 104–105, 283

peripheral neuropathy, 105, 283

personal trainers, 33–34, 188

pharmacist, 32–33, 283

phentermine/topiramate ER (Qsymia), 76

physical activity, 283–284. *See also* exercise

physical exams, at checkups, 44

physician assistants (PAs), 26, 284

Pilates, 185

pills, for type 2 diabetes, 57–63

pioglitazone (Actos), 58, 61, 284

PMS (premenstrual syndrome/symptoms), 112, 113

pneumococcal pneumonia vaccines, 42

podiatrist, 34–35, 284

polycystic ovary syndrome (PCOS), 114

polydipsia, 284

polyphagia, 284

polyunsaturated fats, 144, 284

polyuria, 284

port lights, on blood glucose meter, 86

portion control, 159, 162, 284

portion size, 159, 163

positive actions, 202

positive thinking, 202, 256

postmenopause, 118

postprandial, 284

potassium, 149, 150

PPSV23 vaccine, 42

pramlintide (Symlin), 63, 64, 284

prediabetes, 13, 14, 15, 59, 215, 284

preeclampsia, 12, 20, 114

preferred provider organization (PPO), 284

pregnancy

  cautions for women with preexisting type 2 diabetes, 13

  cautions with some type 2 diabetes medications during, 57

  cautions with weight loss medication during, 76

  considering your eyes during, 263

  delivery, 117

  guidelines for healthy pregnancy, 20

  healthy mom, healthy baby, 113–118

  planning for, 114

  postpartum, 117

  qualifying for CHIP, 233

  taking care of yourself and your baby during, 114–116

  for teens with type 2 diabetes, 220

  weight loss after, 118

premenstrual syndrome/symptoms (PMS), 112, 113

premixed analog insulin, 68

premixed combinations of short- and intermediate-acting insulin, 67

premixed insulin, 68, 69, 284

preprandial, 285

prescription assistance programs, 236

progesterone, 112

progress, measurement of, 46

progressive disease, 225

proliferative retinopathy, 261, 285

proteins, 137, 143–144, 285

proteinuria, 285

psychiatrist, 35, 285

psychologist, 285

Q

questions and concerns, making time for at checkups, 43

Quick Diabetic Recipes For Dummies, 171, 208

R

RACCs (reference amounts customarily consumed), 160

race, as risk factor, 15, 215, 264

random plasma glucose test, 14, 15, 285

rapid-acting insulin, 73, 181, 285

rebound hyperglycemia, 285

recipes, 171, 208, 209

Recognized Diabetes Education Program, 285

Recommended Dietary Allowance (RDA), 285

reference amounts customarily consumed (RACCs), 160

registered dietitian nutritionist (RDN), 31, 132, 285

registered dietitian (RD), 31, 132

registered nurse (RN), 285

regular insulin
  defined, 286
  Humulin R, 68
  Novolin R, 68

Rehabilitation Act of 1973, 243, 245

repaglinide (Prandin), 58, 60, 286

repetition (in exercise), defined, 184

resistance exercise, 183–184

restaurants, 174, 175. *See also* eating out with confidence

retinopathy, 101, 286

rights, knowing yours, 241–249

risk factors, 15–16, 264, 286

rosiglitazone (Avandia), 58, 61, 286

roux-en Y gastric bypass, 77

Rule of 15, 93–94, 286

Rx Outreach, 237

S

saccharin (Sweet'N Low, Sugar Twin), 142, 286

safe sex, for teens with type 2 diabetes, 220

safety guidelines while driving, 249

salt, a little goes a long way, 151

saturated fats, 145, 146, 150, 286

saxagliptin (Onglyza), 58, 60, 286

SBC (Summary of Benefits of Coverage), 230

SC (subcutaneous), 287

secondary diabetes, 286

sedentary lifestyle, 286

self-care routine, 49, 107–108

self-monitoring of blood glucose (SMBG), 286

serum creatinine (eFGR), 41, 44

serving size, 147, 148, 159–160, 161, 168, 169, 170, 171, 175, 286

set (of repetitions), defined, 184

70% aspart proteamine/30% aspart (Novolog Mix 70/30), 68

70% NPH/30% regular
  Humulin 70/30, 68
  Novolin 70/30, 68

75% lispro protamine (NPL)/25% lispro (Humalog Mix 75/25/), 68

sexual activity, for teens with type 2 diabetes, 220

sexual discomfort, during menopause, 121

sexual health, 109, 210

SGLT2 (sodium-glucose cotransporter 2) inhibitors, 58, 60–61, 287

shingles (Zoster) vaccine, 42, 43

shopdiabetes.org (website), 166, 170, 171, 174, 238

shopping smart (for healthy meals), 171–172

short-acting human insulin (regular insulin), 67, 68

short-acting insulin, 286

Simplefill, 236

simvastatin (Zocor), 75

sitagliptin (Januvia), 58, 60, 286

The Six O'Clock Scramble Meal Planner, 208

skilled nursing facility, 239

skin, 35, 100, 248

skin infections, as often occurring on feet, 103

sleep apnea, 98, 218

sleep trackers, 190

Small Business Health Options Program (SHOP), 231

SMART goals, 182

SMBG (self-monitoring of blood glucose), 286

smokefree.gov (website), 261

smoking, 16, 75, 261

snacks, 172–174, 248

social worker, 36

soda, 152

sodium, 149, 150, 151, 287

sodium-glucose cotransporter 2 (SGLT2) inhibitors, 58, 60–61, 287

soluble fiber, 287

sorbitol, 287

special occasions, celebrating of, 176

specialists, 30–36

split mixed dose, 287

spouses, tips for, 209–211

standard blood glucose meters, 85

starch, 287

starchy vegetables, 139

statins, 75

stevia (PureVia, Stevia in the Raw, Sun Crystals, SweetLeaf, Truvia), 142

steviol glycoside, 287

strength training, 183, 287

stress
  coping with/managing of, 107–108, 196–198
  for teens with type 2 diabetes, 219

stretching, 185, 187

stroke, 11, 19, 41, 49, 64, 65, 74, 75, 95, 97, 98, 99, 122, 127, 144, 145, 164, 178, 224, 226

subcutaneous (SC), 287

subcutaneous tissue, 71

sucralose (Splenda), 142, 287

sucrose, 287

sugar, 141–142, 222. *See also* added sugars

sugar alcohol, 224, 287

sugar substitutes, 142, 287

sugar-free foods, cautions with, 224

sulfonylureas, 58, 59, 288

Summary of Benefits of Coverage (SBC), 230

sunscreen, 248

supplements, cautions with, 57, 151

support
  for caregivers, spouses, and family members, 211
  finding of, 22
  getting of from friends and family to achieve fitness goals, 189
  getting of, giving of, 205–211

support groups, 21, 201–202

surgery, 76–77, 238

sweets, myth of people with diabetes not able to eat, 222–223

synthetic human insulin, 66

syringes, for injecting insulin, 69, 70

systolic blood pressure, 11, 40, 74

T

tai chi, 185

targets. *See also* goals; targets
  blood glucose targets, 13, 18, 20, 30, 38, 39, 56, 82, 83–84, 90, 98, 100, 101, 102, 103, 104, 106, 109, 113, 114, 115, 116, 121, 124, 162, 163, 167, 176, 200, 219, 226, 259, 260
  for blood lipids, 127
  for blood pressure and cholesterol, 40–41, 121
  for heart rate, 186

Tdap (whooping cough, diphtheria, tetanus) vaccine, 42, 43

tea, 152

team management, 288

teens, raising of with type 2 diabetes, 213–220

teeth, 33, 44, 101

telemedicine, 288

test strips, 88

testosterone, tackling problem of low testosterone, 126

thiazide diuretic, 288

thiazide-like diuretics, 75

thiazolidinediones (TZDs), 58, 61, 288

thirst, satisfying of, 152–153

thoughts, minding of, 35

tobacco, 16, 197, 220

Tolerable Upper Intake Level (UL), 288

tonometry, 262

tracking method, choosing of, 89

trans fats, 145, 146, 150, 288

Transportation Security Administration (TSA), 241, 247, 248

travel, planning ahead for, 247–248

TRICARE, 233

triglycerides
consequences of, 41, 75
defined, 288
as risk factor, 16
testing of, 44

TxAssist, 236

type 1 diabetes (T1DM, T1D)
defined, 288
described, 11

type 2 diabetes (T2DM, T2D)
defined, 288–289
as most common type of diabetes, 11
as progressive disease, 225

TZDs (thiazolidinediones), 58, 61, 288

U

UK Prospective Diabetes Study, 19

ulcers, protecting feet from, 103

uninsured, finding help for people who don't have insurance, 236–237

unit of insulin, 289

unsaturated fats, 144

urine albumin-to-creatinine ratio, 41, 44, 107

urine testing, 289

urologist, 126, 289

U.S. Department of Agriculture (USDA), 136, 137

U.S. Department of Health and Human Services, 231

U.S. Department of Veterans Affairs, 231, 233

V

vaccinations, 42–43, 289

Varicella (chicken pox) vaccine, 42, 43

vegetable juices, 152

vegetables, 138–139

vertical sleeve gastrectomy, 77

very-low-density lipoprotein (VLDL) cholesterol, 289

V-Go insulin pump, 73

Viagara, 125

videos, for fun ways to work out, 255–256

vildagliptin (Galvus), 289

vision, taking care of, 101–102. *See also* eyes

VISION USA, 236

vitamin B12 deficiency, 59

vitamin D, 149, 150, 151

vitamins, best sources of, 151

VLDL (very-low-density lipoprotein) cholesterol, 289

volunteering to help someone else, 257

W

waist circumference, 289

walking, as exercise, 180, 255

warming up (for exercise), 185, 186

Warshaw, Hope (author)
Eat Out, Eat Well, 174

water, as best choice if you're thirsty, 152

weight
  effect of metabolism on, 179
  paying attention to, 39, 40
weight loss
  benefits of, 11, 75
  medications for, 76
weight-loss surgery, 76
whole grains, 139–140, 289
wholesome foods, benefits of, 11
whooping cough, diphtheria, tetanus (Tdap)
    vaccine, 42, 43
wine, 153. *See also* alcohol
women
  alcohol consumption, 153, 197
  being mindful of menstrual cycles, 112–113
  focusing on your heart, 122
  healthy mom, healthy baby, 113–118
  hot flashes, 120
  menopause, 118–121
  night sweats, 120

sexual discomfort during menopause, 121
and type 2 diabetes, 111–122
yeast infections, 120–121
working out (for exercise), 185, 186–187
workplace, diabetes in, 242–245

X
xylitol, 289

Y
yeast infections, 120
yoga, 185
yourself
  taking care of, 17–20
  taking time for, 203
YouTube, for exercise videos, 256

Z
Zoster (shingles) vaccine, 42, 43

About the Author

The American Diabetes Association is the nation's leading nonprofit organization fighting diabetes and its consequences. The Association's mission is to prevent and cure diabetes and to improve the lives of all people affected by diabetes. We work toward this mission by funding research to prevent, cure, and manage all types of diabetes; providing services to people and communities affected by diabetes and reliable information to patients and healthcare providers; and advocating for the rights of people with diabetes. For more information, please visit www.diabetes.org or call 1-800-DIABETES (1-800-342-2383).

Acknowledgments

The American Diabetes Association would like to acknowledge Kate Ruder for her tireless efforts bringing this book to life. Thank you for your dedication to creating a reader-friendly, comprehensive guide to all aspects of life with type 2 diabetes. We'd also like to thank Tracy Boggier, Senior Acquisitions Editor at Wiley, and Vicki Adang, of Mark My Words Editorial Services, LLC, for managing this project, as well as Elizabeth Kuball for her thorough editorial work. This book would not have been possible without all of your support, guidance, excellent ideas, and hard work.

Publisher's Acknowledgments

Senior Acquisitions Editor: Tracy Boggier

Project Editor: Elizabeth Kuball

Copy Editor: Elizabeth Kuball

Production Editor: Tamilmani Varadharaj

Cover Image: © Piotr Adamowicz/iStockphoto

Special Help: Victoria M. Adang

Take dummies with you everywhere you go!

Whether you are excited about e-books, want more from the web, must have your mobile apps, or are swept up in social media, dummies makes everything easier.

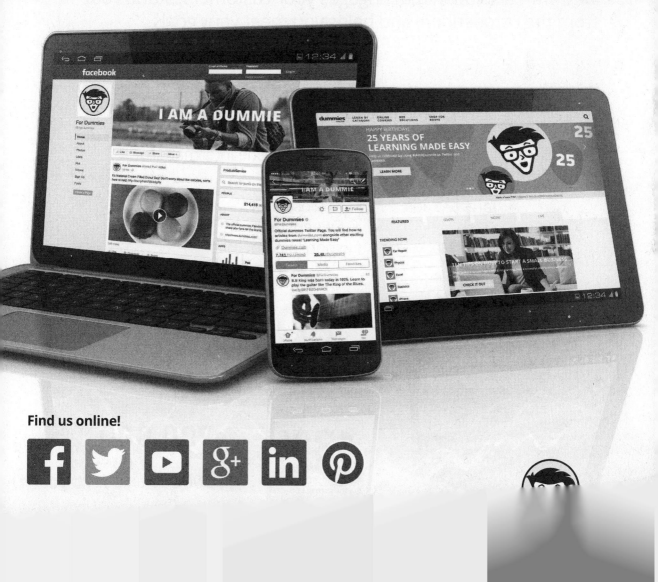

Find us online!

Leverage the power

Dummies is the global leader in the reference category and one of the most trusted and highly regarded brands in the world. No longer just focused on books, customers now have access to the dummies content they need in the format they want. Together we'll craft a solution that engages your customers, stands out from the competition, and helps you meet your goals.

Advertising & Sponsorships

Connect with an engaged audience on a powerful multimedia site, and position your message alongside expert how-to content. Dummies.com is a one-stop shop for free, online information and know-how curated by a team of experts.

- Targeted ads
- Video
- Email Marketing

- Microsites
- Sweepstakes sponsorship

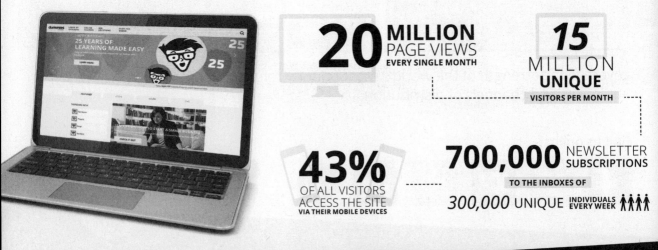

20 MILLION PAGE VIEWS EVERY SINGLE MONTH

15 MILLION UNIQUE VISITORS PER MONTH

43% OF ALL VISITORS ACCESS THE SITE VIA THEIR MOBILE DEVICES

700,000 NEWSLETTER SUBSCRIPTIONS TO THE INBOXES OF *300,000* UNIQUE INDIVIDUALS EVERY WEEK

# of dummies

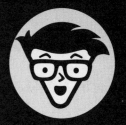

Custom Publishing

Reach a global audience in any language by creating a solution that will differentiate you from competitors, amplify your message, and encourage customers to make a buying decision.

- Apps
- Books
- eBooks
- Video
- Audio
- Webinars

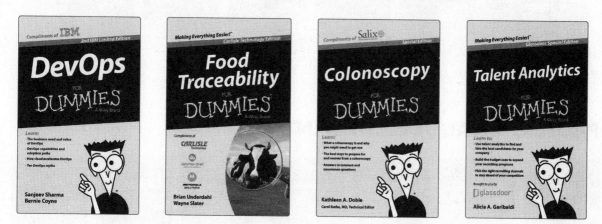

Brand Licensing & Content

Leverage the strength of the world's most popular reference brand to reach new audiences and channels of distribution.

For more information, visit dummies.com/biz

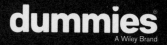

PERSONAL ENRICHMENT

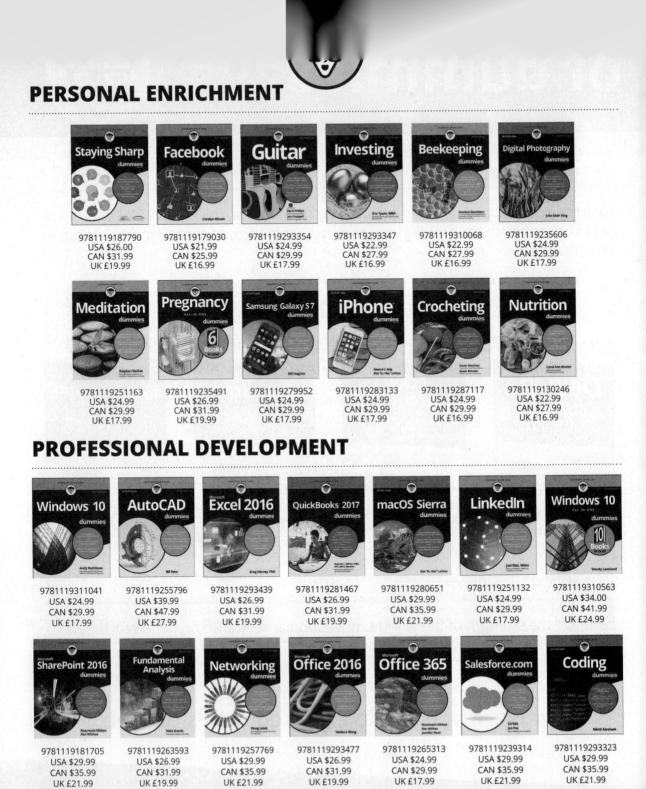

Staying Sharp
9781119187790
USA $26.00
CAN $31.99
UK £19.99

Facebook
9781119179030
USA $21.99
CAN $25.99
UK £16.99

Guitar
9781119293354
USA $24.99
CAN $29.99
UK £17.99

Investing
9781119293347
USA $22.99
CAN $27.99
UK £16.99

Beekeeping
9781119310068
USA $22.99
CAN $27.99
UK £16.99

Digital Photography
9781119235606
USA $24.99
CAN $29.99
UK £17.99

Meditation
9781119251163
USA $24.99
CAN $29.99
UK £17.99

Pregnancy
9781119235491
USA $26.99
CAN $31.99
UK £19.99

Samsung Galaxy S7
9781119279952
USA $24.99
CAN $29.99
UK £17.99

iPhone
9781119283133
USA $24.99
CAN $29.99
UK £17.99

Crocheting
9781119287117
USA $24.99
CAN $29.99
UK £16.99

Nutrition
9781119130246
USA $22.99
CAN $27.99
UK £16.99

PROFESSIONAL DEVELOPMENT

Windows 10
9781119311041
USA $24.99
CAN $29.99
UK £17.99

AutoCAD
9781119255796
USA $39.99
CAN $47.99
UK £27.99

Excel 2016
9781119293439
USA $26.99
CAN $31.99
UK £19.99

QuickBooks 2017
9781119281467
USA $26.99
CAN $31.99
UK £19.99

macOS Sierra
9781119280651
USA $29.99
CAN $35.99
UK £21.99

LinkedIn
9781119251132
USA $24.99
CAN $29.99
UK £17.99

Windows 10
9781119310563
USA $34.00
CAN $41.99
UK £24.99

SharePoint 2016
9781119181705
USA $29.99
CAN $35.99
UK £21.99

Fundamental Analysis
9781119263593
USA $26.99
CAN $31.99
UK £19.99

Networking
9781119257769
USA $29.99
CAN $35.99
UK £21.99

Office 2016
9781119293477
USA $26.99
CAN $31.99
UK £19.99

Office 365
9781119265313
USA $24.99
CAN $29.99
UK £17.99

Salesforce.com
9781119239314
USA $29.99
CAN $35.99
UK £21.99

Coding
9781119293323
USA $29.99
CAN $35.99
UK £21.99

dummies.com

dummies
A Wiley Brand

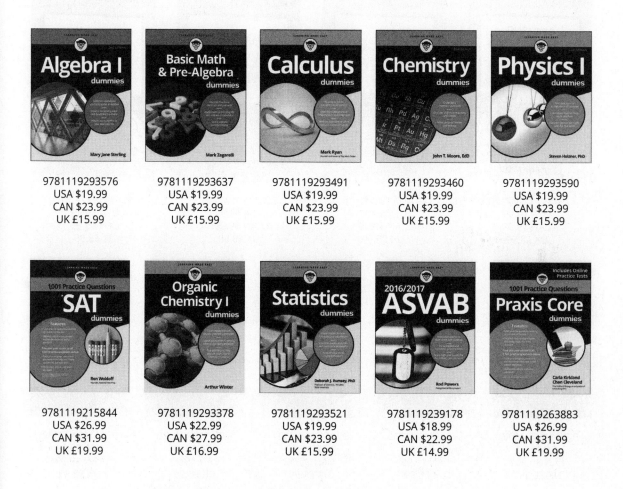
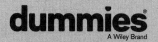

Small books for big imaginations

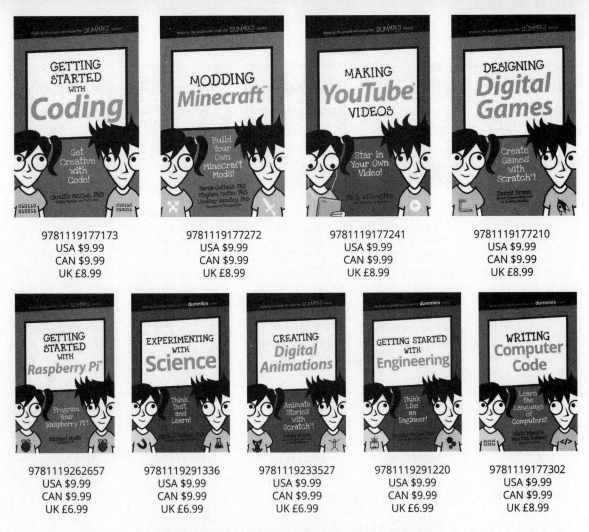

GETTING STARTED WITH **Coding**
Get Creative with Code!
Camille McCue, PhD
9781119177173
USA $9.99
CAN $9.99
UK £8.99

MODDING **Minecraft**
Build Your Own Minecraft Mods!
Sarah Guthals, PhD
Stephen Foster, PhD
Lindsey Handley, PhD
9781119177272
USA $9.99
CAN $9.99
UK £8.99

MAKING **YouTube** VIDEOS
Star in Your Own Video!
Nick Willoughby
9781119177241
USA $9.99
CAN $9.99
UK £8.99

DESIGNING **Digital Games**
Create Games with Scratch!
Derek Breen
9781119177210
USA $9.99
CAN $9.99
UK £8.99

GETTING STARTED WITH **Raspberry Pi**
Program Your Raspberry Pi!
Richard Wentk
9781119262657
USA $9.99
CAN $9.99
UK £6.99

EXPERIMENTING WITH **Science**
Think, Test, and Learn!
9781119291336
USA $9.99
CAN $9.99
UK £6.99

CREATING **Digital Animations**
Animate Stories with Scratch!
9781119233527
USA $9.99
CAN $9.99
UK £6.99

GETTING STARTED WITH **Engineering**
Think Like an Engineer!
9781119291220
USA $9.99
CAN $9.99
UK £6.99

WRITING **Computer Code**
Learn the Language of Computers!
Chris Minnick and Eva Holland
9781119177302
USA $9.99
CAN $9.99
UK £8.99

Unleash Their Creativity

dummies.com

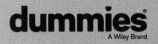

dummies
A Wiley Brand